OVERCOMING MIGRAINE

A practical guide that you can use to heal
yourself, change yourself, free yourself

M. MORE

To my life partner, Vitor,
who was with me on this long road!

To my wonderful parents, Luzia and Jeronymo (who unfortunately is no longer with us), who instilled in me the hunger for reading which unveiled a world of wonders and knowledge for me!!!

To my two dear children, Igor and Lukas, who during part of their childhood had the misfortune of having a sick mother and yet they became such beautiful and blessed beings!

TABLE OF CONTENTS

INTRODUCTION

My principal objective for writing this book is to help people who suffer from pain or chronic illnesses. Cure is possible. It takes time, perseverance and experimentation to find out what works for you.

I will try to be as brief as possible in describing the various paths I took, until I was finally able to heal myself from the chronic pain I had suffered for 14 years. I healed myself, and if I could, you can too!

The purpose of writing this book is not for me to talk about my years of migraine, or asthma, or the various other problems I've had. On the contrary, I want you to focus on finding the perfect health as I did pursuing my cure. But I want you to know that I can talk about pain, I went through all the stages. I did all the treatments I'd heard of. I went to all kind of physicians, Eastern practices, spiritist centers. I tried all the medicines, from the established to the experimental ones. I tried all diets I was told would help, and yet life closed around me and I became a prisoner of the pain. I was in pain every day. I woke up and went to bed in pain. The medicines no longer worked. By the end of those 14 years I no longer recognized myself. Sometimes I cried because I thought I could never ever be again the person I once was. I was so afraid that all that constant pain would eventually cause permanent damage to my brain. Luckily it did not!

It was the worsening of my situation that made me decide that I had to heal myself, because I couldn't go further down. I had to have my life back.

Do you know the horse's lesson? It is an Eastern parable.

It is said that a farmer, who struggled with many difficulties, had some horses to help in the work of his farm. One day the foreman brought word that one of his horses had fallen into an abandoned old ditch. The hole was too deep and it would be difficult to get the animal out. The farmer evaluated the situation and made sure the horse was alive. But because of the difficulty and the high cost of removing it from the bottom of the pit, he decided that it was not worth investing in such resources.

He summoned the foreman and ordered him to sacrifice the animal by burying him there. The overseer summoned some of the servants and directed them to throw sand on the horse until it was fully covered and the pit offered no more danger to the other animals. However, as the sand fell on his back, the horse would jerk and knock it down and step on it.

Soon the men realized that the animal was not letting himself be buried., but, on the contrary, it was rising as the sand fell; until finally it was able to leave.

Like the horse, I was at the bottom of the well, and I felt that the world was trying to bury me forever. The last physicians I went to simply gave up on me. Literally, they told me that there was nothing else they could do to help me and that I should get used to living that way. No kidding! That was my ultimatum, get used to it or give up living entirely. Undeceived by the doctors, I realized that I was going to have to find a solution on my own. I know now that their giving up was the best thing that happened to me in a long time. I decided that I would heal myself no matter what. And now I am healed!

When you make a decision it's amazing how the universe leads you towards what you want. Soon after making that decision, several videos and books began to appear. Everything I needed to know to be able to heal myself was just showing up. I was changing habits, changing my mind, controlling my thoughts, cultivating the certainty that I would succeed. I am sure that my journey will serve as an example and hope for you who are reading this book. You can heal your life, we all can, and if you're waiting for a sign, THIS IS YOUR SIGN. Start now, at this very moment. Do not delay. Decide that you will heal, regardless of the difficulties or how discouraged and hopeless you are or have been. Decide now that, despite any setback, you will persevere, because it is perseverance and determination that leads to victory. It's an arduous journey, but the prize is unmatched. Perfect health! I got it! You can too!

Last remark: As the proposal for this book is to be practical, I will separate them into small blocks that can be read randomly, in whichever way you prefer.

GUIDELINES

Here's what you're going to do to heal yourself. You will sign a contract with yourself stipulating that you will follow the guidelines in this book for at least 30 days. Yes... get a sheet of paper and write, "I, So-and-so, decide that I will follow the guidelines of this book, without question, for 30 days and I will heal myself". Date and sign.

Why do you need to do this? There are two main reasons. The first one is that I 'm telling you to do it, I, a person who has healed by following these same guidelines. Think with me ... You've been trying to heal yourself so far and you have not been able to. Then someone who was once at the exact same place you are now, comes up with a recipe for success, telling you what to do. Wouldn't you think it's at least worth a try? After all, you only have two options. Do what anyone who has overcome the problem did or keep doing the same things you have been doing expecting a different outcome? No comments. Perhaps this is the biggest problem I have ever noticed in my life observing the human being: expecting different results always making the same choices. This is never going to happen. For something to change, you need to change first.

The second reason is that the brain has a different way of processing the facts that most of us still do not understand. It defines its reality through fragments that it captures from the environment and catalogs according to the knowledge it has accumulated throughout its life. Let me give you an example: You left home today with a swollen right eye because you have an allergy. You looked at yourself in the mirror before you left and thought you looked like you had been punched in the eye. You arrived at the office and while sitting at your desk, you see two colleagues of yours drinking coffee and whispering and laughing, looking at you. What your brain tells you is that they're laughing at you because they think you've been punched in the eye. You are absolutely sure that this is what they are whispering and you feel bad about it. Later you learn that your colleagues were looking at you and talking because they knew you were going to be promoted. Your brain told you what it thinks is true, not what is true.

Did you understand what I wanted you to grasp? Reality is nothing more than what your subconscious interprets from the data it captures in the environment. It picks up the data from the environment through its senses, vision, touch, etc., interrelates with what already exists inside you and shows you the conclusion it arrived at. Since the brain does not distinguish what is "real" from the imagination, any more resources you use to reaffirm what you want will add up within yourself and cause the subconscious to build that reality for you. It sounds kind of complicated at first, but as you read on that subject, all the pieces will fit together and you will understand perfectly how to work with your subconscious mind. That's why visualization is a very efficient resource. As your brain does not distinguish between reality and imagination, when visualizing you will be using multiple senses to shape what you want, causing your subconscious to take a deeper record of what are you seeking.

So, make the contract with yourself, in a formal, written way. This will make your subconscious interpret your decision as important, changing the impact of recording that within you.

Below is a short guide on what you have to do to achieve what you want.

GUIDE:

1- You will decide that you will heal;
2- You will create your mantra and repeat it untiringly;
3- You will be aware of the signs that appear around you. There is no coincidence! They will begin to appear; videos, books, etc., that will point you in the right direction.
4- You will stop listening to what others say is possible or not (even yourself, if necessary!). You will create your own set of beliefs based on what you want for yourself;
5- You will introduce physical exercises into your daily routine;
6- You will change your diet. You will introduce good foods and gradually remove inflammatory foods like gluten and dairy products. You will exchange sugar and refined salt for its whole versions. You will decrease the amount of 'sugar' you eat. You will reduce food deficits with supplementation;
7- You will stop taking analgesics and anti-inflammatories;
8- You will block thoughts about your chronic illness (or any other problem you have and want to change) and how miserable you are for having it;
9- You will walk the road of personal development reading books, watching videos, etc.
10- You will introduce some relaxation practice into your routine, whether listening to videos with binaural sounds or meditating;
11- You will focus solely and exclusively on what you want - perfect health (or whatever you want to change/achieve). Every time your subconscious mind takes you to another focus you will redirect it back to perfect health. You control your thoughts, you control your emotions, you control your body. Write it down on a piece of paper and carry it with you until it turns into a belief deeply rooted in your subconscious.
12- Persevere! One step at a time. Do not think about what is still missing. Focus only on today and now, which is the only moment you have total control. What can you do today? Never give up. Persevere!

By following these guidelines, you will achieve everything you want in life. I'm sure! In the next blocks I will clarify several points covered in this guide and more. I will say it again: you can do it!

Block 1

"Lost time is not recoverable. Make sense of your life now!"

M. More

DECIDE

At first seems silly to have a topic like this. Surely everyone wants to heal. The thing is, it's not that simple and I'll explain why.

Between wanting and deciding there is an immense distance. If you look inside your mind, you will find a lot of "I want" and very few "I decide" and why? Because when you give the command - I decide - everything is different, your whole brain/mind/emotions/thoughts structure themselves differently; they act distinctly. Take a practical test, stop for a moment and talk to yourself, "I want to lose 2 pounds this month," "I'd like to ..." and then say, "I decide to lose two pounds this month." Did you notice the different feelings that your brain sent you?

When you want to change something in your life you must decide to do it. A decision makes your brain/mind/spirit have a goal to follow. It's as if you give a command "well, I'm here now and I want to get there, what should I do next?" And the answer comes, you can be sure of that.

I'll make an analogy of what the decision does in your life. Your life is like a ship in the sea adrift. It can berth at any port, but you will only be able to reach a specific place if you have a route to follow. Your decision, what you want, is the route to follow. So, you must decide what you want, in all aspects of your life, only then can you achieve your goals. You need to know what you want for yourself in relation to all important things to you such as health, life goals, relationships, wealth. If you do not know where you want to go, life will take you anywhere, and maybe it will be a place you wouldn't like to be in, the ocean is a vast place to adrift.

Take some time and think about the important aspects of your life and what you want for yourself. Then write it down! Understand that your brain processes reality through your senses and the more senses you use when deciding on your goal, the more areas of your brain will be activated and more records will be made. Taking these actions make them to become more and more real to your brain and consequently for yourself. What you think becomes real.

Decide now, at this very moment, that you will have the perfect health, that you will heal. I made that decision two years ago and within a few months my life had totally changed. When I look at who I was then and who I am today, it seems a miracle that I have attained, not only in relation to my health, but in all areas of my life. This achievement is due to deciding and changing the words inside me, focusing my thoughts only on what I wanted.

Pause now and write on paper that you decide to have the perfect health, a wonderful relationship, wealth, and everything else you want. Do not simply ask for what you think is possible ... ASK FOR WHAT YOU REALLY WANT!

Persevere, No Matter What!

"THE PATH OF DREAMS TO SUCCESS EXISTS.
MAY YOU HAVE THE VISION TO MEET IT,
THE COURAGE TO REACH IT,
AND THE PERSEVERANCE TO FOLLOW IT."

KALPANA CHAWLA

There is not much to talk about on this topic, despite its importance. You simply need to persevere always. There is no way to achieve anything without perseverance, without determination. You need to internalize the "baby lesson": try, fall, get up, go on, walk ... Have you ever wondered what would happen if a baby gave up trying to walk? If he had looked at those dumb little legs and thought, "I'll never be able to do that?" What did the baby do? He persevered. Baby lesson: no matter how many times I have to try, my goal is to walk!!!! First the baby decided to walk, then came the means, the muscles, etc. This is how you should go on in life, with patience and perseverance, having a goal to achieve.

Every time you feel weak, sit down, inhale deeply and try to rescue the childlike tenacity within you. It's there, somewhere, waiting to be fed. Think of everything you have achieved to this day, despite the difficulties and how great it was the sense of triumph for having succeeded. If you are so negative about yourself now that you cannot think of anything, go farther. Think about when you were little, how difficult it was to walk, talk, ride a bike, overcome the fear of sleeping alone, make that tangle of letters become a story. Do not trivialize a child's achievements, they are amazing and are there to encourage us to move on despite the difficulties.

Other lessons from children: "Create Borders, No Limits," "Trust Your Instinct, It Is Your Best Guide," "Do not Let Fear Hold You from Trying," "Do not Waste Your Time with rocks in your head, the empty mind is capable of performing inspired miracles," and so on.

The easiness and amenities we have in our present life are inspired miracles. A miracle is nothing more than a fact that human contemporary knowledge has no ability to explain. Imagine yourself coming back in time for your great- grandfather and telling him that you will call him via skype, that he will see you moving in real time, etc ... Do you think he would have the ability to understand? Of course not, that would be a miracle to him. Do not be limited by what you think is impossible today.

All the great advances of mankind occurred

when a simple man went beyond the limiting

barrier of the possible and created the impossible.

Make a little book or a board of miracles with real and desired achievements. Hang it in a place you can always see for those times when you need extra cheer you up. Do not think that achievements are only social ones like employment, home, car... If today you are a better human being than yesterday, this is conquest. In fact, this is the greatest achievement you can desire: be happy regardless of anything.

PARABLE OF THE ANT

The other day, I saw an ant carrying a huge leaf. The ant was small and the leaf was at least ten times the size of it. The ant carried it with perseverance. Sometimes it was dragging it, sometimes it had it on his head. When the wind beat, the leaf fell, causing the ant to fall as well. There were many obstacles, but the ant did not despair over its task.

I watched it and followed it, until it came near a hole, which should be the door of its house. That's when I thought, "At last the ant finished its journey."

My illusion.

In fact, it had only completed one stage. The leaf was much larger than the mouth of the anthill, which caused the ant to leave it outside and then enter alone. That's when I said to myself, "Poor thing, so much sacrifice for nothing." I also remembered the popular saying, "Swam, swam and died on the beach."

But the little ant surprised me. From the hole came other ants, which began to cut the leaf into small pieces.

They seemed cheerful in the task. Before long, the large leaf had disappeared, giving way to small pieces and they were all inside the hole.

Immediately I found myself thinking about my experience. How often did I get discouraged by the size of the tasks or difficulties? Maybe if the ant had looked at the size of the leaf, it would not even have begun to carry it.

I envied the persistence and strength of that little ant. After my encounter with that ant, I came out stronger in my walk. I thanked the Lord for putting that ant in my path or for making me go through it.

FAITH

For me this is another simple topic. We either have faith or give up living. I approach faith in the same way as other intangible matters, I do not argue about it. Is it better for me to have faith? Is my life happier, fuller? So, I have faith and nourish this feeling inside of me because I want to be happier and fulfilled. Without faith, there is no way we can live in this world. Even though some have an easier life than others, we all go through situations that take us down and make us want to jump on the train of life. What holds us is faith. I'm not talking about religion; I'm talking about FAITH. Faith, by itself, is something far above and deeper than religion. No matter how you cultivate it, whether it's part of a religion or not, you must cultivate it in the truest way for you. I do not think that faith is an easy thing to explain, nor do I propose to do so, but I think we all carry this feeling, to a greater or lesser degree. It is this feeling that urges us to go on, to hope that things will change for the better. Faith makes us feel confident that there is meaning to life and suffering. The more faith you have, the happier you are and the easier it is to live.

Do you know the parable of the farmer who planted corn? When asked by a student about what religion was, he replied:

> – *"Oh, you lad," said the old farmer, "to me, religion is just like my corn harvest here in my land."*

> – *"Corn harvest?" the student asked for an explanation.*

> – *"Well, let's see. The people who live here in these lands prepare the soil, choose the seeds, plant them, fertilize them, take care of*

them until the time of the harvest ...but after this, you have to bring the harvest to the city market to sell it. To get there, we can go by either of three paths. There is the old dirt road path, there is the path of the river of the meadow and there is the path of asphalt road. But then, when we arrive there in the city and there sell our produce to retailers, they won't ask about the path that lead us there. They will want to know if the corn is good."

There are various ways of cultivating faith, e.g.: by being part of some form of religion, realizing the magnitude of the perfection of the universe in which we live and how it could only have been created by a higher being/beings, practicing meditation, listening videos with binaural sounds and subliminal messages about connection with the universal source of wisdom, or use EFT. I used EFT a lot when my father passed away. I was in a state where I could barely breathe, feeling so much pain that seemed physical and moving on then was practically impossible. The only idea that came to my mind at that time was to use EFT and even without believing it would work in this case, I did it. I used phrases to increase my faith and belief, that I was still going to see my father, that he had not simply disappeared, etc. Over the days and weeks that followed, the pain was relieved, I got back to being functional, I believed that I would be happy again and I succeeded.

To finalize, I would like to reiterate that cultivate faith is something essential for a happy and full life. Do not belittle its importance.

Use What You Learn

To use what you learn seems so obvious that I almost did not add this topic in the book. However, after thinking about the comprehensiveness of this simple attitude I decided to include it.

There are a lot of people who read, study, dialogue and even teach, but when you take a closer look at these people's lives, you realize that they are limited to this. They have never implemented anything they have learned, and if you do not do it, I'm sorry, but you're not going anywhere. So... USE EVERYTHING YOU LEARN (good things, of course!). Only then you will know what works or not for you. As an example, I can cite EFT. When I started using it, I felt retarded hitting the technical points, but even then, and even with a certain disbelief, I did not give up. I use this technique to this day and I have already taught it to several people. Some of them have used the technique and some have not, but this is not my concern. Each person has the free will to decide their own life. I do what I think is right for me and passing on the knowledge I gained through a troubled life is important to me.

As the parable says, *"the shepherd takes the sheeps to the water, but it is up to them to drink or not."*

So, I'll repeat try! The battle can be big, but never, at any moment of your life prefer the previous defeat to the possibility of the victory. Never waste the opportunity to get what you want. If you have to put yourself upside down blowing a whistle and eating watermelon to get it... What are you waiting for? Try, try, try, until you find out what works for you.

STAY TUNED

When you ask God or your Higher Self for something, when you decide to do something, the whole universe goes on with you in this journey. Things will start to show up for you and you need to be aware of them. Someone will say a phrase that it will bring you an idea, or a thought, you will watch a video showing you exactly what you needed to know, a book tip, it does not matter how it comes, it will come and you need to realize and take action about it. Do you know that joke of the believer?

During a great flood that occurred, a very religious man did not leave his house at all. When the water reached his feet, a man in a canoe passed by and invited him to board, and he replied:

– No thank you. God will save me.

When the water was already in his waist, two young men came in a boat offering help. And the answer was the same:

– I do not want your help. God will save me.

As the water reached the believer's neck, a helicopter passed by rescuing the last people, and someone shouted for the man to grab the rope to save his life. And again the stubborn replied:

–I do not need it. God will save me.

But the water rose and the man drowned. He came to heaven and soon complained to God,

–Gee, I trusted You, my Lord. Why did you let me die?

And God answered,

–My son, I sent you a canoe, a boat, and a helicopter, what else did you want me to do?"

Most people are like this believer, blind to the situations around them, as much as obvious they are. That's why I decided to explore this topic. I know how sometimes we do not pay attention to the situations around us. We are so absorbed in ourselves and our problems that we lose the opportunities that appear. There's a technique I always use when I ask for something: I ask to be able to realize what it is been sent to me, or that I be able to understand the answer. So, here's the tip - always be aware and if you are too obtuse, ask for focus and the ability to see.

Mantras

Translating from Sanskrit, mantra means 'instrument of thought' and thinking you can change your world, as I have changed mine.

"Your strongest beliefs were

tranquil thoughts one day."

I am totally adept at focusing on thoughts that express the changes you want to achieve. In so many books, it is said that you must change your vibrations to achieve what you want, but until you change the vibrations there is a way to go, which is sometimes left out of these books.

The first step in achieving any change is to change the "words" that you say to yourself. At the root of all your problems are the beliefs that you created in some moment in your life and perpetuated with the phrases that are constantly being said. You need to pay attention to what you say to yourself and modify any recurring negative thinking. Even not believing at first! Understand: first comes words, then changes. For example, if you want to be more confident you need to stop self-deprecation and say things like: "I feel extremely confident in every situation, I know my values and I feel wonderful when I express my opinions." To be braver and face situations that make you anxious and uncomfortable like a job interview, tell yourself on the way to the interview: "I am powerful and command all my emotions. I am always in charge of myself, I always feel super calm and know exactly what to say. I radiate extreme confidence. People always realize how extremely confident and capable I am. I`m a lovably person." Do you understand the concept? You need to tell yourself how you want to feel, to behave, how you want people to perceive you. With the constant repetition of these new ideas, they will become familiar to you and will be incorporated by your subconscious as a standard. One tip is to always use hyperbolic, exaggerated words. These words make your unconscious give a greater sense of importance to the phrase.

Now you must create your phrase/mantra by stating what you want. Here is the mantra I created to find the path of my healing: 'My health is perfect, my head is always good and I always feel extremely well.' I constantly repeated this mantra, feeling well or not. I got to a point where it was repeated in my head even unconsciously. My brain got used to constant repetition and created this habit to make my life easier, probably the point when things started to change.

Nowadays, I can easily change the vibrations I feel, but when I started this journey, I could not. When you are plunged into a bad situation, you can hardly change your vibrations, so one of the tools that can help you change them is to create your mantra and repeat it relentlessly. A phrase that works and makes sense to you, that your brain does not reject.

What will happen is that over time, new thoughts, circumstances, books, videos, will begin to appear guiding you in the direction of your desire. When you consciously think about a subject, you feed it, and the more you focus on it, the more you intensify its vibration. It's like starting to study anything, at first you're not very good, you do not get it right, but over time, the accumulation of information increases and, if you want, you can become an expert. Initially your thought is just a point in the intricate sea of thoughts you carry, but by constantly focusing your attention on that particular thought, you are forming a new drawing. Every drawing starts with a dot, have you thought about it? From a small point, you can draw anything you want.

In my case, the first significant thing that appeared was the video "What the Bleep Do We Know !?"

(https://www.youtube.com/watch?v=R6G3-Zc9mtM&t=43s)

After that came out the book Super Brain, by Deepak Chopra and Rudolph Tanzi. It was this book that produced the click, my "eureka", that changed my life. This book made me realize thoroughly that the brain is a being of habits. After this acknowledgement I just had to link the dots... I was born sick, all my life I was sick! So... how could my brain produce health without knowing what it was? I always had an illness because my brain didn't know what it is to be healthy. Never, in this life, there was a healthy me. Because of that, as you can imagine, it was difficult to change. I had to train my brain to change decades of a single habit – to be sick. But I did, and the difficulties that I passed through become small because of the gift I received - health! If I was able to convince my brain, my body, to be healthy, I, that was born sick, you can do it too.

You need to create your mantra and do not be discouraged.

Each person has their time. Each person is at a different stage in life. My path may not necessarily be yours, but it will give you ideas of where to begin, what to try, and the Wisdom Source will direct you to exactly what you need to know, hear, or read. The most important thing is to not give up, to continue, to believe, to have faith.

This technique of creating your mantra can be used in any area of your life. Wealth, success, love, inner peace, self-confidence, no matter what you want to change in your life, this can be your beginning. You can start wherever you want. If you do not believe in the laws of the universe and even if there is an infinite source of well-being, you can start there. How about, "I am always filled with an immense confidence and a certainty that everything will be ok in my life!", "I am extremely happy and grateful for the immense faith and trust I have in the Wisdom Source", "I am very happy and I always feel very good!". Choose what works for you.

A great way to starting on your path is by increasing your faith and confidence, because the more you believe, the easier it is to manipulate the energy field around you and attract the things you want.

Demystifying Physicians and Social Paradigms

"Never allow any book or person to overlap your judgment. A book is meant to teach, instruct or even entertain.
A book is not a master to be followed blindly or without reason. No person gifted with intelligence should be left enslaved by a book or the words of another."

Lama Mingyar Dondup

Being a physician, priest, pastor, or whoever, does not make anyone more than just a human being, with his faults, vanities and qualities. To heal yourself, you need to understand that. Medicine is not and will never be an exact science as some tend to affirm. Doctors make decisions based on what they've studied, what the medical board sanctions, what colleagues in the profession use, what common sense says, and so on. Worst of all, the current occidental medicine, for the most part, is based on illness, not on health.

Just because a physician said does not mean that it is real. It is only real to him, with the baggage that he accumulated in his experience. To explain what I want to say, I will tell you what happened to me. The year I decided to heal myself, three doctors, of different specialties and even different nationalities, told me that I would have to learn to live with migraine. One of them still tried to give me hope by saying that maybe, at menopause, there would be some improvement. One of the neurologists told me that there was nothing else he could do for me. I had already tried all the treatments available. The other one asked me if I wanted to start over again one of the treatments that I had already tried to see if it would work in that point. I guess I just did not jump off a bridge after hearing these "formidable" prognoses because my experience had already shown me that the truth of a person, regardless of who it is, is no more than that – the truth of that person in question. These prognoses only made me realize more deeply that I was going to have to do it myself.

This is a necessary requirement for healing: build a mindset of your own, regardless of traditional methods or what is believed to be the truth. Be sure there is always an answer and a solution to any problem. Your healing exists, you just need to find it, inside or outside of you.

Stop Taking So Much Medicine

My life turned to shit, pardon my language, because the first neurologist I went to, told me: At the first sign of migraine, take the cocktail (analgesic, anti-inflammatory, antiemetic), and if you are not ok in an hour, repeat them. In my ignorance on the subject, I did exactly what he told me to do. With that attitude, over the years, the frequency of migraines increased. The intensity decreased a little and after 10 years of constant worsening, my pain became daily and not very intense. Do not think that the pain being milder is better than having debilitating crises a few times. IT IS NOT!!! The daily pain ruins your life, undermines your resistance and changes you more than sporadic episodes.

If you have not yet reached this stage, do not take pain medication unless it leaves you in bed or vomiting when you move. Take analgesic or anti-inflammatory only in extreme cases. If you think I'm being too drastic, do some research. Look into the effects that the prolonged use of analgesics and anti-inflammatories cause both in your illness and in your body as a whole. I wish someone had told me that years ago, it would have saved me a lot of suffering.

Make yourself aware that you are addicted to analgesics, that you depend on them both physically and psychologically. Perhaps this is not so clear in your mind, so I'll give you an example of another incurable disease that I had, asthma, which shows this addiction pretty well. Whenever I traveled, I carried my inhalator and the medicines with me in case I had a crisis. I was once traveling with my boyfriend through the countryside, on vacation, when at the end of the day the weather got gloomy, heavy clouds appeared in the sky and it became totally dark. We passed a sign announcing a city. I told my boyfriend that we should sleep in this city because it would still take about four hours to reach our destination. We entered the road and after a while we arrived at the edge of a river where there were several cars parked. We discovered that the town we were headed to was, in fact, an island whose only access was in a kind of canoe. So far so good, adventure! It was already raining, we were tired, so we decided to stay right there. When we disembarked on the other side of the river, we learned that there was no electricity on the island, only power generators, but they were turned off at 10pm. This information made me very nervous because, without electricity, if I had a crisis, I could die. I wanted to leave. I was already feeling my breathing change, my lungs tightening. My boyfriend convinced me, due to the horrible weather, to talk to the hotel owner to see if there was anything he could do. The owner of the hotel was very supportive and calmed me down saying that there was a generator that I could use if I needed. Instantly I felt the soothing substances released by my brain circulate throughout my body, my lungs began to decompress and the onset of crisis was gone.

As you can tell, in addition to physical dependence, I had total emotional dependence as well. I was fine until I knew there was no electricity. From the moment the fear appeared, the beginning of crisis came along and my breathing became difficult. This case reveals two important facts. One is that we become emotional addicts of substances that "heal" us. The other fact is that any disease has an underlying emotional background. Think and reflect on this, "no disease is only in the physical". Understanding this is the key to your cure. Try to read about it. It is an important milestone in the solution of any disease.

It Happened To Me

Now I will tell you what happened to me when I decided to stop taking medicine. You will realize why it is so important to make the decision to heal yourself, because if you are not firm in your decision, the obstacles that appear will bring you down.

I took analgesic, anti-inflammatory and antiemetic almost every day for a long time. To be honest, they didn't really stop my pain anymore. I was totally dependent on these medications. However, from the moment I discovered that it had been the painkillers that got me to that point, I decided not to take them anymore. I simply stopped. After deciding to heal me, that was the most important step I took.

The craving to take the medicines was immense, and even though I knew they were no longer making my pain go away and, on the contrary, they were making my pain continuous, I still wanted to take. The chemical and emotional dependence was great. I was able to spend 20 whole days without taking any medicine, a stupendous victory for me, which gave me more confidence that I could heal. To my surprise, and joy, the daily pains were dwindling as early as the first month. After a while, the symptoms I had experienced in the beginning of dealing with migraine were coming back when they appeared two to three times a month. The crises were horrible. Sometimes I could not even move. I experienced heavy nausea and pain in my whole body. These crises were so intense and incapacitated me in such a way that my husband had to stay with me at home to help me. But understand this, those horrible crises were my brain wanting me to take medicine so it could continue to live in the same way. The famous terror barrier! It was its way of trying to make me go back to what it was used to. And it is in this moment that you will need more willpower. This is the time when you will tell your brain that you are the one who is in charge and, from that moment on, you will never take pain medicine again and it will have to accept your decision and change. Because the boss is you and now you have decided that your health is perfect and you will have to find a way to make it happen. Do you understand? The brain will do anything to keep a habit, be it good or bad for you. You need to stand firm in your decision and know that this phase will pass and you will be able to have the perfect health you seek. You need to focus on the outcome you are looking for.

I decided that those crises were synonyms of improvement. They were sporadic, increasingly sporadic. Over time, and with my determination to continue detoxing, they passed. Today, I no longer have these crises. Sometimes I do get headaches, but like any normal person, it's a pain that passes!

Another thing that happened to me was that in the first 2 months of detox, I started having insomnia. I would wake up and not be able to sleep throughout the night. I even went to see the doctor about this. He gave me a sleeping pill that I used twice. I thought to myself "Oops, I just got rid of an addiction, will I get another one?!" I decided that phase would pass and it did. Today I sleep much better than I slept in those 14 years I suffered from migraine.

If you go through this, there are several alternatives that can help you not involving medicines. Try natural alternatives such as magnesium (mainly magnesium malate), floral, melatonin, teas, meditation, isochronic and binaural sounds, magnetic bracelet with FIR, germanium and ions, etc. In this phase I also discovered that playing games like Tetris, Candy Crush, Farm Heroes and so on, made me sleepy and it was what helped me. Sounds unbelievable but it is true! Recent discoveries have shown that the conscious mind does not have the ability to process two things at the same time and because of the constant visual appeal and the need to perform small tasks in these games, any agitation or problem in your mind disappears while playing, allowing you relax. There are studies on this subject worth reading. I reassure you; your cure depends on only you. Whatever your illness or problem, there is a solution. So, research, study, change

BLOCK 2

"THERE IS NO PUNISHMENT OR REWARD,
WHAT EXISTS IS CONSEQUENCE.
PLANTING IS FREE, BUT HARVESTING IS MANDATORY."

BIBLE

CHANGE YOUR LIFESTYLE: NUTRITION

Before getting into this topic, I want to make it clear that despite accumulating years of study in this field, I do not advocate the right to prescribe anything to anyone. It is up to each one to research and decide what is best for themselves. I learned early on to use my own judgment to decide what is best for me. I also learned that it is not because it is written, or because people say it, regardless of who, that makes a fact to be true or not. The truth of yesterday is not the same as today, which will not be the same as tomorrow! So, my advice, start to use your own judgment to decide what is best for you.

There is a lot to talk about in terms of nutrition. However, since the purpose of this book is to be concise, I will not delve into it. It is therefore up to you to seek this knowledge. Always remember that it is you who must take care of your health. The information nowadays is democratic, it is there for those who want to learn, it is available regardless of any social or financial criteria.

I also want to emphasize that if you decide to take supplements, there is a very clear rule to follow: do not look for price, look for quality. Always research on the credibility of the brand and read the label to be sure of what you are buying. Try to read about the substance you have decided to take and the correct formulation to be well absorbed by the body. You can always look for a good integrative medicine specialist, if you prefer.

Regarding nutrition Dr. Jerry Tennant, founder of The Tennant Institute for Integrative Medicine, says:

"The process of rebuilding a new and healthy you is based on the fact that the body is constantly replacing itself. Your body grows new retinal macular cells every two days, new skin in six weeks, a new liver in eight weeks, and new nerve cells in eight months. As each new cell is built, the body seeks proper building materials from which to construct the cell. If the body cannot find good, healthy materials, it will use whatever is available."

So, nutrition is the key to a healthy body.

As general rule, I believe that it is important to cut industrialized products out of your diet as much as possible. Drastically reduce sugar consumption and have a varied, preferably organic, natural diet. In addition, supplementing with essential substances that are lacking in food, due to several factors, among them, the impoverishment of the soil.

Those who have a chronic disease certainly have nutritional problems. Be it the disease that has caused the deficiency or vice versa. The sick person, more than all others, needs to be aware that he must have a healthy diet, take supplements, do physical and mental exercises, get into a good sleep routine, and adopt a positive attitude. You will not be able to heal yourself until you start to walk this path.

Several things can be the chronic pain cause such as a simple food allergy, a mineral deficiency, jaw problems, hormonal problem, some fracture poorly cured, and the list does not end. If you are reading this book, probably you already did a thorough search. In this chapter I will stick to nutrition.

You need to do experiments with yourself. There are certain substances that are part of almost everyone daily diet that are highly allergenic such as gluten and milk products. To see whether you are allergic or not, try cutting these and other substances. Cut out gluten for at least a month, if nothing improves, cut milk and dairy products, or everything together. If still there is any improvement, cut out red meat. Trial and error. You will eventually find out what works well for you.

There are several types of diets, for various types of problems; ketogenic diet, blood type diet, fodmap, etc. You, who have some "incurable" disease, need to try all the alternatives until you find the one that works for you.

It may be that your problem is not in what you eat but in what you are failing to ingest. Here are some essential substances for good health (besides sleeping well, of course!) that is missing in the diet of most people:

- Water of good quality;

- Integral salt – coarse salt, pink salt, etc.;

- Vitamin D3;

- Magnesium;

- Iodine;

- Omega 3;

- Vitamin K2;

- Iron;

- Vitamin B complex.

Not to mention countless other substances that you may be lacking.

Over the years, the reserve or the production of certain substances by the body decreases. Deterioration by use intensifies, which can cause various health problems. "Aging" (encompassing a whole paradigm of physical and senile illnesses here) today, must be regarded as a consequence, not the cause of the diseases connected with the third age. Nutritional deficiencies and a very strong archetype "of the elderly" intensifies a whole process that could be much slower. Not to mention that science has overtaken this story that the older person loses intellectual capacity. Just research and you will find extensive material regarding it. In fact, you do not even have to use science to prove it. Think about it, how many elderly people do you know who has incredible mental capacity?! Perfect health? Who has more energy than some younger people?

What I see happening is people limiting themselves to this paradigm of old age and allowing themselves to grow old. If you forget something when you're 30s, you're tired and you do not even give a shit about it. But if at 70s you forget; you, and most of the people around you, will think you're getting senile. Maybe Alzheimer! Isn't it absurd? I've seen this happen several times. This discussion about aging is very long and out of the main focus of this book. But one thing I want you to store in your mind: aging is not synonymous of illness and disability. Nowadays aging with health, disposition and energy is a matter of choice. This is a very interesting subject to study. Read about brain plasticity and epigenetic. Knowledge modifies you. It makes you evolve. Study!

Returning to the subject of nutrition. There are also substances that can help improve health and can be used together or separately:

- Turmeric;

- Coconut oil;

- Alpha lipoic acid;

- Coenzyme Q10;

- LDN (low dosage of naltrexone);

- Collagen;

- Astaxanthin;

- Berberine.

To be in perfect health, you must also follow some parasite elimination protocol such as that of Dr. Clark or Kroeger Herbs. There are others besides these, just search about it. There are several studies on this subject that show how parasites affect our health and are not detected by normal tests. Studies also say that most people are contaminated and do not even know.

GOOD QUALITY WATER

People are dehydrated and do not even know it. Water is the most important nutrient (yes, a nutrient) for the human body and, in general, people give very little importance to it. If you think that, on average, 70% of your body is composed of water and it is absolutely central to every function of each cell - whether it's muscle contraction, cells dividing, or nerves conducting, etc., it is not difficult to reach the conclusion that it is the most essential substance for our survival! Here is a figure showing the average percentage of water in the various organs of your body:

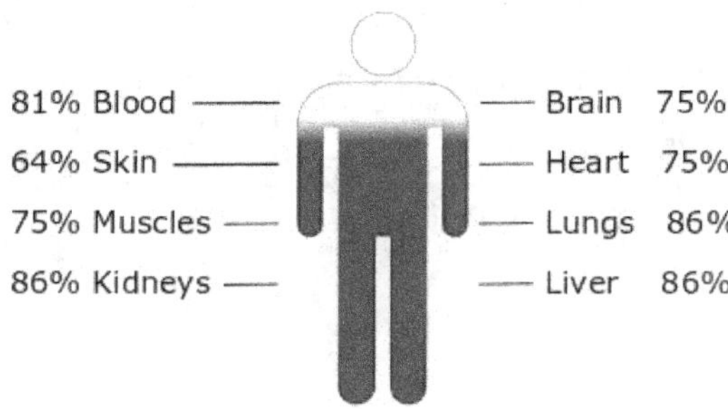

Below is another figure showing how we dehydrate as we age.

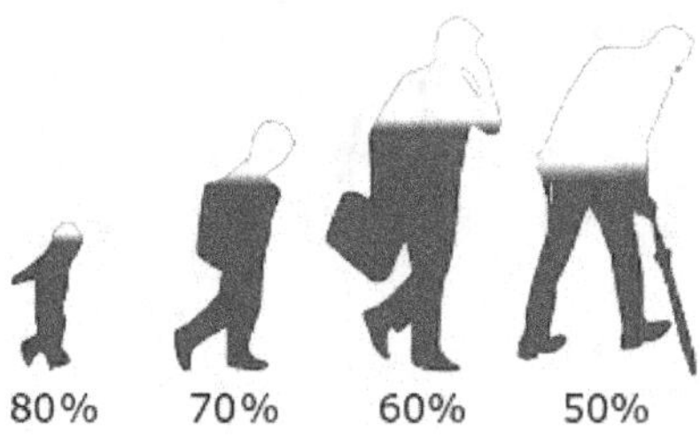

It provides us enough material to think, doesn't it? Water vs. aging? Getting sick? How about instead of spending alarming sums on products to rejuvenate the skin you invest in a quality filter and rejuvenate the entire body?

Water deficiency manifests itself rapidly: a variation of about 1% in the degree of hydration already leads to the appearance of the symptoms of dehydration.

An adult need to drink, on average, 8 glasses of water per day. You can add a pinch of whole salt to your water to mineralize it because, if you developed a chronic dehydration over the years, just tap water can solve your problem. If you are the type who forgets to drink water, drink more glasses every time you drink, or walk with a bottle.

Here's a warning, bottled water is not necessarily good water. Various parameters such as the distance from the source to the final consumer, PH, redox, etc, come into question here. You should invest in a good filter. But research well before you buy.

If you would like to know more about the importance of the water and what type of water you should be taken to really hydrate your body, there are some books really good like "Cells, Gels and the Engines of Life"– Dr. Gerald Pollack.

VITAMIN D

Vitamin D is a hormone that is synthesized in humans following skin exposure to ultraviolet B radiation. It regulates the expression of hundreds of genes, participating decisively in the functioning of various organs and systems of the body. Its lack leads to a myriad of problems, from simple daily disturbances like fatigue and pain, to life-threatening illnesses such as diabetes, heart disease and cancer. Its deficiency is related to several other pathologies like asthma, osteoporosis, rickets, atopic dermatitis, multiple sclerosis, inflammatory bowel disease, rheumatoid arthritis and even depression.

Like it was said, the sun is the main stimulus for producing vitamin D in the body and more than 80% should come in that way. The big problem is the generalized heliophobia. Nowadays people flee from the sun as if it is a villain. If not only that, they soak up sunscreen in such a way that the sun cannot reach the skin directly. Without sun, there is little vitamin D.

If you search in the internet you will see that a big part of the world's population is deficient of this vitamin. Even in tropical countries you will find very high statistics. The maxim that the sun is bad must have been created by the industries that sell sunscreen. The worst thing is that you do not even have to dig deep to realize the lack of foundation for this dictum. I'm not saying here that you should spend a whole day at the beach without sunscreen, but you need to absorb sunlight directly into your skin, preferably between 12:00 and 14:00hrs, for a few minutes a day and take vitamin D3 supplements if necessary. You must research on sunscreens before buying. Not all contain protection against UVA rays, the radius that reaches the Earth all day.

MAGNESIUM

Magnesium is responsible for more than 350 biochemical reactions in the human body, including energy generation, protein production, muscle movement and nervous system regulation. The list of direct and confirmed disorders with chronic or acute deficiency of magnesium is long. Unfortunately, a large part of the world's population does not get the necessary amount of magnesium, and traditional medicine does not solve that insufficiency. That's because nutritional therapy is not taught in most of the medical school. Magnesium is not considered as a therapeutic agent in hospitals or doctor's offices and is not a patentable drug. For all these reasons, conventional medicine remains blind to the extent of magnesium deficiency and potentiality.

Magnesium can help treat heart problems, chronic pain, chronic fatigue, fibromyalgia, migraines, anxiety, premenstrual syndromes, osteoporosis, hypertension, insomnia, and so many more health-related issues.

I've been taking magnesium for a long time. Since starting, I've felt much better overall. The main benefit I noticed was the quality of my sleep. In addition to promoting deeper sleep, it also reduced my need to urinate at night. Also, when I feel a slight headache, in addition to the capsule of turmeric, I take magnesium. Even for fever, I discovered recently, magnesium is efficient. A month ago, I got the flu, which is an unusual occurrence for me, and I had a low fever. As my body was sore, I decided to take magnesium. Besides improving the pain in my body, after a while, my fever subsided. Without further remedy!

You find magnesium in various formulations like magnesium chloride (poor absorption), magnesium malate (the best for the heart, because of malic acid, which I use), magnesium L-threonate (better for the brain), magnesium glycine (for the bones), among others. Read about it and decide which is best for you.

IODINE

Iodine is one of the most important minerals for the proper functioning of the body. It is imperative for the production of thyroid hormones, which regulate our metabolism, the absorption of minerals among many other functions. In addition, it is important also for the adrenal glands, ovaries prostate, breasts. In short, it is needed throughout our endocrine system. Iodine is also a powerful detoxifying, chelating and germicidal agent. It eliminates toxic metals and chemicals, facilitating the immune system's service.

Iodine deficiency is one of the most common nutrient deficiencies. According to the World Health Organization (WHO), a third of the world's population suffers from some problem related to the deficiency of this mineral. This is due to several factors, including the lack of iodine sources in the diet and the constant exposure to the antagonists of this mineral. Iodine is part of the halogen metal group as well as chlorine, fluorine and bromine, and they compete with each other for absorption. Unfortunately, in the actual world, we are exposed to an absurd amount of these metals, which are highly toxic to the human body alone and, if not enough, also decrease the absorption of the little iodine we ingest.

Summarizing, people do not ingest iodine enough to enjoy all the benefits it brings or even to supply the body. The Lugol solution can be purchased from any drugstore and is extremely cheap.

OMEGA 3

Omega-3 fatty acids are essential for many bodily functions. They are not synthesized by the body and because of that, they are obtained either through diet or supplementation. Among the extraordinary benefits that it brings are:

- Helps to improve joint pain and stiffness;

- Helps reduce inflammation;

- Improves brain capacity and memory;

- Helps strengthen the immune and nervous systems;

- Promotes healthy eyes, skin and hair;

- Improves overall health and mood;

- Decreases triglycerides levels;

- Helps lower blood pressure;

- Helps prevent degenerative brain diseases;

- Prevention and amelioration of autoimmune diseases;

- Improves sleep quality.

VITAMIN K2

Until recently, vitamin K2 was not known, it was just vitamin K. There is now an impressive amount of research showing that vitamin K2 plays a very important role in human health, ensuring that our bones grow strong and that our hearts and blood vessels remain healthy.

One of the important functions of vitamin K2 is to direct the calcium ingested by the body to the bones, thus preventing calcium from being deposited in the wrong places such as arteries, joints and organs, which could cause arteriosclerosis, arthrosis, kidney stones, calculus vesicular, cataract, etc.

Among the sources of vitamin K2 are fatty meat, liver, tongue, heart, but mainly of grass feed animals. It is also found in egg yolks. Other source is fermented food like natto and miso, common in some eastern countries.

TURMERIC

From the first time I read that turmeric was considered the most potent and natural anti-inflammatory in the world, I decided it was going to be part of my diet. It was one of the first additions in my daily diet that produced improvement in my migraine. Until recently, I bought the natural turmeric from an Indian market near my house. Now I'm taking capsules from a manufacturer that certifies 95% of curcuminoids, which is the part of turmeric that science proves gives the results. I think it really is more potent, because after I started taking that turmeric, my overall health is a way better. Recently, my son was having headaches because he started using braces. From the first day of taking turmeric his headaches just stopped.

Anyway, let's look closer at this wonderful seasoning, not in flavor, because I definitely do not like it, but for health...

Turmeric is, besides a powerful anti-inflammatory, a potent antioxidant. It also increases the levels of brain-derived neurotrophic factor (BDNF), which is the protein responsible for the maintenance of established neurons. Besides that, it allows the growth and differentiation of new neurons and synapses. In summary, it can help prevent and even reverse problems in the brain. It's great for the stomach as well. It's worth incorporating it into your diet.

ALPHA LIPOIC ACID

Alpha lipoic acid is a powerful antioxidant. It is produced in small quantities in the human body and, like numerous other substances, its concentration decreases with aging.

Among the many benefits it brings are:

-   improves the absorption of sugars;

-   improves diabetes-related neuropathies;

-   restores body energy levels;

-   prevents aging by its antioxidant action;

-   helps liver regeneration;

-   decreases fat liver;

-   helps improve vision and prevent cataracts.

Alpha-lipoic acid has been called nature's ultimate antioxidant because, among other things, it is fat and water soluble and recycles various substances in the body like Vitamin C, Vitamin E, Coenzyme Q10 and also glutathione.

If you want to know more about alpha-lipoic acid there are several very good books like Alpha Lipoic Acid Breakthrough - Dr. Burt Berkson. Dr. Berkson also has several videos talking about his successful experience in treating various forms of cancer and autoimmune diseases with low-dose naltrexone (LDN) and alpha-lipoic acid.

COENZYME Q10

Coenzyme Q10 is a substance also synthesized by the human body itself and is vital to produce energy. Many medical studies show benefits of coenzyme Q10 when taken as a supplement, most of which results from its vital role in oxygen utilization and energy production, particularly in cardiac muscle cells.

Coenzyme Q10 is beneficial to the heart in many ways. It helps maintain the normal oxidative state of LDL cholesterol, helps to ensure circulatory health and supports the optimal functioning of heart muscle. In addition, coenzyme Q10 helps reduce and decrease the severity of migraines.

For those who use statins, it is essential to replace coenzyme Q10, because statins block the production of this coenzyme which is fundamental for the heart. Is it not absurd? The medicine that was supposed to help, in most of the cases causes more harm than good. I think I've heard this story before.

LDN

LDN - low dose of naltrexone. Naltrexone was initially approved at high dosages (50-300mg) for use by narcotics dependents because it acts by neutralizing the opioid system, in other words, it prevents the drug addict from being high.

Naltrexone in low dosages blocks the opioid system only for a short time, causing the human body to react by manufacturing various endorphins, which regulate cell growth, and their respective receptors, optimizing and enhancing the body's immune system.

The main benefit of this body response to LDN is a decrease in inflammatory processes in the whole body, an increase in the immune system and chronic pain decreasing in general.

LDN has been successfully used in the treatment of various types of cancer, including pancreatic, autoimmune diseases such as Crohn's disease, chronic fatigue syndrome, Hashimoto's thyroiditis, fibromyalgia, degenerative diseases such as Parkinson's, Alzheimer's, etc. The list keeps growing because its applicability is immense.

WHOLE SALT

In the last decades salt was turned into a villain, and what is incredible is the number of people who believe in this lie. It's one more of these absurdities that the media and people are spreading without even clarifying the facts. Table salt, refined, is heavily processed to eliminate minerals and usually contains additives to prevent clumping, but whole sea salt is a true polymineral. It contains traces of more than 80 minerals. Today, with the impoverishment of the soil, more than ever, it is necessary to use salt to get minerals.

Salt is a vital substance to keep the body hydrated. It helps maintain the electrolyte level necessary for the proper functioning of the organs, supplying various minerals like magnesium, calcium, potassium and sodium.

Electrolytes have many important functions in your body; among them, they regulate your heart rate and enable your muscles to contract so you can move. Sea salt can help prevent an electrolyte imbalance, which can cause all kinds of severe symptoms.

CHANGE YOUR LIFESTYLE: EXERCISE

"LIFE IS LIKE RIDING A BICYCLE.
TO KEEP YOUR BALANCE, YOU MUST KEEP MOVING."

ALBERT EINSTEIN

Here are 7 reasons to exercise regularly:

- Releases endorphins in the body, making you feel happier;

- Strengthens the muscles and consequently the bones;

- Increases the body's energy levels;

- Helps reduce the risk of chronic diseases;

- Leaves skin more beautiful;

- Increases your logic capacity;

- Improves sleep.

There are many benefits that introducing exercises into your daily routine brings to your life, these are just a few of them.

I think most people fail to introduce exercise into their everyday routines because they have too many paradigms. They have learned at some time in their lives, that to get out of the zone of sedentarism you have to do at least 30 minutes of daily exercise for at least 5 days a week, or 1hr, 3 times a week, or that they are too fat, or too skinny, or too old, and think that is it or nothing. It`s not quite right. Get it all out of your head. You need to be aware that ANY exercise is better than none. Always! Regardless your age or body proportion, you will benefit from exercise. Time, that great villain, can also be your big ally, because time passes by and exercising becomes easier. Your body will adapt to the new routine and, make no mistake, once you acquire this habit, your body will want more.

The best way to create a daily routine, be it exercising or any other habit you want to acquire, is to create goals that you are sure to achieve. An example; you want to get in the habit of work out, but you always do not have time enough, energy, or any other excuse of the kind. You will then commit to take 5 jumps every day, or park the car further away from work, or use the stairs instead of the elevator. Do you understand the concept? You create a goal so small that you will reach regardless of any situation. In fulfilling your goal, you will be creating within yourself the vibration of "I get". Whatever you do beyond your goal will be an extra. Want to create the habit of reading? How about one page a day? Over time, once you get into the habit, extending your goals becomes a lot easier.

To extend this subject "create a habit/change a habit", how about reading some books on the subject? I assure you that learning about how the brain works will change your life. The best book I read on this subject was the Super Brain by Deepak Chopra and Rudolph Tanzi. This was the best for me because it was the book that woke me up to understand the brain as a being of habits. However, there are many others talking about the same subject, such as The Power of Habit by Charles Duhigg and Mini Habits by Stephen Guise.

If you're lazy to read a book, buy an audiobook, listen on the way to work, school, while cooking, anywhere! Do not create obstacles for your growth, create shortcuts. Make your life easier.

CHANGE YOUR LIFESTYLE: MIND/SPIRIT

"EVERYTHING IS ENERGY AND THAT'S ALL THERE IS TO IT.
MATCH THE FREQUENCY OF THE REALITY YOU WANT AND
YOU CANNOT HELP BUT GET THAT REALITY. IT CAN BE NO OTHER WAY. THIS IS NOT
PHILOSOPHY. THIS IS PHYSICS."

ALBERT EINSTEIN

EVOLVE

We are here on Earth to evolve! This is an axiom that you should incorporate into your life because if you are not moving forward, you are walking backwards. Nothing is static in life. This is one of the universal laws you must learn.

To be truly happy, prosperous, healthy, confident and have inner peace, there is only one way: to study and to walk towards a goal. A boat that does not have a direction to follow does not get anywhere!

You need to study the laws that govern the universe and, consequently, yourself. The road of self-knowledge leads us to the life we always wish. A life with meaning and accomplishments.

Pause now, close your eyes, take a deep breath and try to hear what your emotions are showing you. One minute, ten seconds, it does not matter! Stop, take a deep breath and turn your attention to yourself. What did you see? Emptiness? Pain? Lack of purpose? Cause I tell you, no matter where you are now, I've been in all these places, even more than once. You have everything you need in yourself right now to change. To have the health you want, the inner peace and the happiness you desire, you just need to walk forward, study and apply what you study in your life.

You can start by taking small steps, no problems. Listen to a video of Bruce Lipton, Bob Proctor, Marisa Peer or start listening to an audiobook when you go to work such as "The Biology of Belief", "The secret", "Think and Grow Rich", "The Power Of Your Subconscious Mind", or something similar. When you take the first steps, the whole universe walks with you, propelling you. You just have to commit to moving on, the way you can, exactly where you are right now. Never give up. Study every day even for just a few minutes, changes come with the assimilation of new concepts and is repeating that you get there.

In Search Of Yourself

Do you know who you are? Not your name or your profession. Who are you really!? If I asked you "who are you?", would you know how to respond? If not, start there, look at yourself and see who you are. Do you like yourself? What would you like to be different? What would you really like to do with your life? The whole journey of self-knowledge begins in ourselves, asking us "who am I?, am I happy?, what do I desire?". Not to judge us, but to know where we are and where we want to go. An essential knowledge to have a better life.

There are things I know about you that you may not know. You are already on the road of evolution. This book is in your hands responding to your appeals. There is no coincidence. What we call coincidence is nothing more than the law of attraction acting in our life.

All these negative emotions we feel are because we moved away from our true essence. As you begin to walk the path of evolution, that connection begins to re-establish itself and, gradually, happiness, abundance, and inner peace begin to return. The great news is, you're already on your way. Continue. Persevere. You can. The power to get everything you want is within you.

HABITS

OSHO

Another thing you need to learn is that we are beings of habits. Your brain has been made to make your life easier. So, as you repeat behaviors and thoughts, your brain becomes familiar with them, and the next time the fact that originated that behavior or thought happens, your brain will respond automatically, more and more efficiently. That rule applies to everything. A great example is to learn to drive. When you start you get tense, your brain is extremely alert and you think of all the actions you need to take; accelerate, brake, look at the rear-view mirror, etc. What happens next? Over time? You enter in your car from your office, arrive at home and you even notice how it happened. Your brain made your life easier; it created a HABIT: to drive, the way you taught it. Is that not fantastic? Does it not open a world of possibilities? You can train your brain to do whatever you want to do. This is an extremely important concept. Stop for a moment and think about it. Assimilate this new knowledge, this is probably the most practical knowledge you will learn to change your life.

Now, think about yourself and everything you do during your day and realize that all your habits have been built through training. How good or bad you are at something is directly related to the time you put into it and the quality of related thoughts. There are very simple and universal examples like: you walk, because you trained until you got it; you talk because you trained; you read, because you trained. Understood? Anything, any habit, that you want to acquire, there is only one way to achieve it, to train/study!

"All you want for your life is,
inevitably, just a training distance!"

The your "selves"

At this very moment, I want you to begin to assimilate the idea that there are three main characters that together form your self: your unconscious/ subconscious/ brain, your conscious/ mind/ you and your Higher Self/ Guardian Angel. This is a new concept that you must internalize and work within. Here is a representative picture so that you better understand what I am talking about:

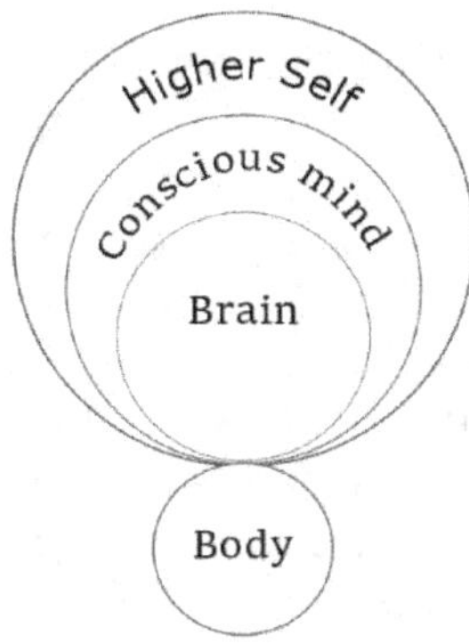

Let's explain it in parts. Your brain/unconscious mind works for you, it is like an employee. You can look at him as the CEO of your company Body Corporations. You are the owner of the company. YOU, who are reading this book. You have a highly skilled employee who manages the company for you. You must give a name to your employee/unconscious mind so you can make a clear distinction between the parts that make up you. By doing so, it will be easier to visualize and make the changes you want. In this example the unconscious will be called Jack. The conscious is yourself, you do not have to give a name, and Higher Self/Guardian Angel/Mana (whatever you prefer to call this superior entity) is going to be Cate. Jack, you and Cate work in synergy.

Going back to the explanation... Jack is a very skilled employee, who solves everything but does not have the ability to see what is best for you. His actions are based on the habits he has learned throughout his/your life and are based on the past. All habits are based on the past! He is a bit of a hardhead and to make him understand and change, you need to teach him the same thing, several times. He only learns with continuous repetition. To change a habit that no longer works for you, you do not attack Jack from the front. Because he is an excellent employee, you build a new habit, a better habit, which makes the old habit unnecessary, as *Buckminster Fuller* explains very well:

"You never change things by fighting the existing

reality. To change something, build a new model that makes the existing

model obsolete."

This process of separating the parts that make up your "selves" makes easier to promote the changes you want, because you can separate what you have created previously and Jack/unconscious mind perpetuate, being an employee of ingrained habits, and what you are creating now. An example: you have changed your thoughts and now you think "my health is perfect" but you continue having headaches. You can look at the situation and see that what is happening is Jack working the way he has learned, not the reality you are creating now. It is not you. Today reflects the thoughts and beliefs you have had in the past.

The more ingrained a belief, the harder it is to change it. But it is possible, you can change anything that you want in you. You just need to be persistent and move forward, have faith and trust. Never give up! Remember the movie's motto "No Retreat, No Surrender!". It is that kind of choice and firmness that you must have.

I will explain the same thing differently because this concept is so important that I think it is worth splitting it in the most diverse possible forms. Understanding this concept changed my life.

Who drives your life in every aspect of it until you "wake up" (learning what I'm explaining to you right now) is your unconscious/brain/Jack my buddy. He has created a set of guidelines for your life which was made up of everything you have learned since you were born and believe to be true. Yes, you think it's true, because the truth to you is nothing more than what you believe to be truth, based on your past experiences, not necessarily on what is real.

Just to you apprehend this very well, I`ll give you some facts. The unconscious mind processes 400 billion bits of information that is around us, but we become aware of only 2000 of those 400,000,000,000 bits. Really!! Where does all the rest go? It remains around you, without you noticing! In logical terms, what this means is that there is a world of realities going on around us that we just do not perceive. And we do not see because Jack only focuses on what he knows, unless YOU set a new focus for him. Seems incredible?

Do you know how you see something? Your brain divides what you see into four components: color, movement, shape and depth. Each of these components is analyzed individually and then compared to the stored memories. Emphasis on stored memories! So, the brain combines all this and shows you what you see. Isn't it an extraordinary fact? It is not only in vision that this happens, the human brain builds our entire reality through associative memories. It relies on the past to create your today. Putting all this together, you realize that the reality that we perceive is nothing more than an interpretation of what it is surrounding us!

Another example: when you were little your brothers always teasing you calling you fat, because they realized that it bothered you and you know how brothers are. You have grown and even though you have never been fat, not even chubby, you are never satisfied with your body. You always think that you need to lose weight, diet, etc. What happened is that you recorded it in your unconscious and as long as you do not realize that is the reason you are always struggling with your weight, you are not going to be happy with yourself. You will always think of yourself as being overweight, whether it's true or not. Because??? Because it's not a question of what's real or not, it's simply a matter of what you think is real!

Getting back to the subject, your unconscious is formed by all your thoughts about yourself, about life, about what you can and cannot do, and so on. How is this way of living is woven? It depends on the age. Until about the age of six, everything that someone said to you to be true will be assimilated as such by your unconscious. In childhood, you have not yet created the barrier between the world and the unconscious, your conscious mind. So, if someone ever calls you dumb, fat, or whatever, this will become true to you. After that age, which can change from person to person, everything that comes from outside is assimilated by the conscious mind, your filter, where it will be decided if it is important, true, consistent with what is already there, so repeated which should only be true, etc. The associations begin.

"Every thought produces a record in the

unconscious, in Jack. And if the repetition of this thought, or subjects

similar to it, is constant, over time,

that thought becomes a habit."

And it is this conscious mind that it is your you that matters. It is you who are reading this book now and learning how to work your mind. Learning that no matter how ingrained a habit, or belief, with perseverance, you can change it. You have just learned that you, and only you, are the master of your destiny. You are the one who looks at a sunny day and thinks "what a beautiful day!". You are the same person who looks at a sunny day and thinks "Wow! It must be so hot that I'm not going anywhere!". Or, "I'll take an umbrella just in case it rains later", or even, "I detest sunny days, only serves to bring more flies!". Do you see the difference? It is you, and only you, that produces your thoughts. You can choose, regardless of the feelings that a day of sun awakens in you, because you are not your feelings, nor your thoughts. You choose them. What you feel today reflects your past. You change your thought patterns today and tomorrow you will be different.

Let's go now talk about the third part of you – your Higher Self, or whatever name you prefer to call. This is the part of yourself that is above you, which is linked directly to universal wisdom and can help you to have the life that you desire more easily. As previously decided, the Higher Self of the example will be Cate. Choose a name that sounds good to you, a name that you feel at ease with.

Anyway, back to Cate. Cate can do anything, whatever you wish for, she can make it happen. It is your particular "Merlin". When you do not know what to do, just say, "Cate, I do not know what to do. I've tried, I've worried about it and I've not gotten anywhere. So, I leave it with you and from now on I will not worry about it anymore. You know exactly the best way to solve this problem and you will either solve it or show me clearly what I should do". Then leave it to her, do not think about it again. Give it a deadline, I want a solution for it by Friday, in 48 hours, 24 hours, it does not matter. Do not think about this problem anymore. This is the only condition: trust that the solution will appear. Over time you are getting good at it, nowadays I'm an ace and I always marvel myself at how it works. I remembered a small example now. The other day I was writing about a certain subject and had only found an example for it and wanted a second to emphasize it. I searched and searched and nothing. I was already frustrated when I remembered "Cate" and I decided to ask for help. I said her I wanted an answer in 15 minutes. I turned my eyes to the page I was already reading and next to it, in bold, there was the call for an article whose title was exactly the question I had asked Cate. Never had my answer been so literal. I do not know if you have already experienced this, but I had that feeling of "full happiness" inside of me, feeling totally in tune with the universe.

This joke of naming "your selves" seems silly, but it is highly effective because one of the biggest problems I noticed is that people find it difficult to see that they are not their thoughts or feelings. They are the entity that created the thoughts, which introduced them into the brain. But you are not them. They don't control you. On the contrary, you can modify them precisely because you created them. This separation brings you power because, ultimately, you see that you can change, that you are bigger and more powerful and can determine what happens in your mind with study, practice and persistence.

Extending this subject, at your side there are several other individuals composed in the same way and with their "Higher Self" connected to yours. Around all these individuals there is another circle, connecting everything and everyone in the universe, which shows us why we are able to affect the people around us and the world, consequently. This is the first universal law – the Law of Divine Unity. Everything and everyone are connected. There is no separation.

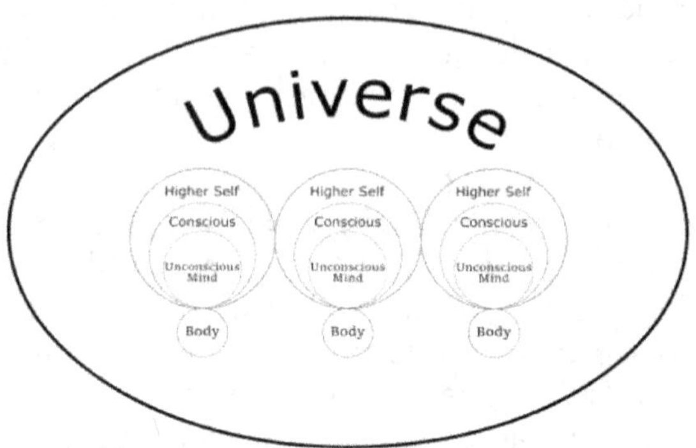

Does it seem like a rather difficult concept to accept? In the beginning it is always like this. There is a certain rejection, because your brain - Jack - has learned differently. But... think for a second.... Re-read this chapter. Even without accepting the concept, start as if it were a joke. Give names to your selves and play with them. As I always say, sometimes you just need to keep the doubts quiet and don't question; just do it.

Learn About the Laws That Rule The Universe

You need to study and study and study, always. Repeat the same concepts until you assimilate them in an indelible way. Read books on the same subject, there is a lot of excellent material available. If you do not want to read books, as I have previously suggested, listen audiobooks, watch videos. No matter how, just seek knowledge constantly, and little is better than nothing, always! Do not impose too many conditions, just do it, every day. By doing what you want to achieve every day, even a little, you open yourself up to a new world. You are training your brain, showing it what matters for you and your subconscious has just one way out; makes whatever you are repeating a habit, a reality for you.

There are several laws that govern our universe and do not think they are laws of any religion or something of the sort. They are laws like the Law of Gravity. There is and that it is all. It is not because it is not possible to see through our eyes that something does not exist. Remember that what you see is simply the result of associative calculations made by your brain. Come on, other examples that are part of our daily life which we not see and we do not think about them? Electricity, internet, radio, television, telephone? We do not see what makes the phone work or how we can talk to someone on the other side of the world in real time over the internet, but even so these things do exist. You can use them without believing and they will still work, because they exist independently of you. Isn't it wonderful to know that? Read the next paragraph keeping this in mind.

To change your life, the most important universal law you must get acquainted with is the Law of Attraction. This law can be explained in this way: you attract to you, to your life, everything that is vibrating according to your energy pattern. Our thoughts, feelings, words and acts produce vibrations which, in turn, attract similar vibrations. Negative energies attract negative energies and positive energies attract positive energies.

The more you become familiar with it, the easier it is to consciously manipulate the law of attraction. Do you have difficulty accepting that we are vibrational beings? Let's think a little about facts already proven by science.

Surely you know our bodies are made up of atoms, right? But did you know that an adult has an average of 7,000,000,000,000,000,000 (7 octillion) of atoms? And that most of these atoms are an empty space and that if you compress a human body it will occupy a very small box? Did you know that the nucleus in relation to the empty part, which is full of energy in fact, is comparable to a fly inside a cathedral? Did you also know that the atoms that make up matter never touch each other? The closer they get, the more repulsion there is among their electric charges. When you sit in a chair you are not actually touching it, your energy field is repelling the energetic field of the chair to maintain the energetic unit of your body. This is not "metaphysical", this is physics, proven. But it seems incredible, doesn't it? You are an electric field. Electric fields emit vibrations and similar vibrations attract each other; did you get it?!

If you look for information about this subject you will find plentiful material that makes it easier to believe in Universal Laws. Do not forget the basic principle of everything, the lack of proof of a fact does not prove that it does not exist. It simply proves that that human being, with their current science, emphasis on "current", does not yet have the necessary capacity to prove it. The Law of Gravity has always existed but was only formulated around 1660 by Isaac Newton.

Think about the greatness of these facts and how much we do not know and do not see?

Summarizing all of this – You are, have, live, exactly the way you designed to the universe. And, just as you have built your 'now', with your past thoughts and actions, you can build your future exactly the way you want, thinking differently in the present.

A WAY FORWARD

"YOUR STRONGEST BELIEFS HAVE ONCE
BEEN QUIET THOUGHTS."

UNKNOWN AUTHOR

My first tip is also the latest discovery I made. It began with the questions that everyone asks themselves when they decide to take the road of evolution:

"How can I change my life if I do not believe I can change?", "How can I use the law of attraction if I think it is a stupid idea?" or, "What's the use of listening to or reading what people like Napoleon Hill, Earl Nightingale and Bob Proctor talk about it if I think it's all balderdash?! Very nice to hear, but it does not work with people like me."

So, I'll tell you something very important. Pay attention! It does not matter!! IT DOES NOT MATTER!!!

You do not have to believe for the Law of Attraction to work. It's a law, like the Law of Gravity, as I have said. Regardless of what you think or believe, it will work. Follow the steps, believing it or not.

"If you think you can or if you think you

cannot, anyway you're right."

Henry Ford

I'll give you an example of what I mean. As I said in the preface, I was cured of a chronic pain that I had suffered for 14 years. Almost completely healed, I still suffered from occasional pain. During this time, I decided to ignore the pain. Do not suffer it in silence as I did at the beginning of my healing process, but simply ignore it. I was talking to myself, to my brain and to my Higher Self:

"This pain does not belong to me anymore, you can stop producing it. This automatic response that you have when I step through certain situations no longer exists. All the synapses and paths that you have created to make it easier for me to have pain are rendered useless, there is no more pain. Now I command you to produce just perfect health in me. All the cells of my body are perfect and, therefore, only produce perfect health."

Not that I said all this all at once, or all the time. But every time the discouragement threatened to grab me, or doubt that I wouldn`t get it, I would never be able to get rid of the migraine, I blocked all these thoughts and repeated, and repeated, and repeated versions of this. Until one day all this became true to me. The phrase "my health is perfect, my head is always good and I always feel very good", was my constant mantra. I repeated it so many times that, in the end, without even realizing it myself, it repeated itself in my head.

From all this, what I want you to understand is that, regardless of what you believe deep down, do not let this stay in your consciousness because, no matter what you believe or not, what is in your consciousness it will be registered in your unconscious, who is the master of habits and beliefs. The unconscious mind (you should name it, as I said, your inner dialogues will be clearer) records EVERYTHING that it is in your conscious mind, and if, in a constant way, you feed the same subject, the vibration related to that subject will be strengthened. Every time you think, speak, act, etc, the vibration is going to grow stronger and stronger until it becomes part of you. In conclusion, control what it is in your conscious mind, choose what you think. It takes some time in the beginning to train yourself but, gradually, like everything in life, it gets better and easier. Probably this it will be the most important learning of your life because when you master your mind you can control your life.

UNIVERSE OF INCLUSION

"ALL THAT WE ARE IS A RESULT OF WHAT WE HAVE THOUGHT."

BUDDHA

We live in a universe of inclusion, saying yes or no to something, anyway you are including it in your reality. For the brain "I do not want to ever have migraines in my life or I want to have migraines" means basically the same thing - pain in your head! Already "I do not want to ever have migraines anymore and I want my head to always be good" are totally different statements for your brain. In one you feed all the circuits connected to migraine, strengthening that belief in your brain. In the other you are creating a new set of beliefs related to your head always being good, and the more you feed that thought, the stronger it gets. When you start to pay attention to anything, at first the vibration is weak, but if you start talking or thinking about it, the vibration is intensifying and, over time, any subject will become a dominant thought, a habit.

I will try to exemplify figuratively. Imagine that this ball below is my brain a few years ago. Since I had migraine for 14 years, imagine how many migraine-related synapses I should have? In the matter of health, there was only one thing in my brain - "pain". This grey area is what I imagine was the area taken by the migraine. As you may have noticed, everything in my life was contaminated by it.

Let's continue. This ball represents my brain three years ago, which was when I started my healing process. From this moment on I totally changed my life, mainly, changing myself and my way of thinking. Nothing happened in a blink of an eye. As you might imagine, it was and it is an ongoing process of personal development.

At that time my thoughts were, "How will I heal from the migraine?" "What the hell! I do not deserve this.", "Why do I have migraine if I'm so positive?". I read everything about migraine, tried everything I read that could help, and so what was I doing wrong? Let me tell you what it was my mistake, I was feeding all the synapses about migraine, strengthening them, expanding them.

When I learned that I should change the focus of my thoughts, everything began to change. I started to study how the brain works, what I should do to change my reality, and I began to apply all of that. My life began to change. It was as if an immense puzzle had finally begun to make sense. As if before that, I was trying to put together a puzzle in which I did not have the image to guide me, which is practically impossible.

From then on, I commenced to create healthy thoughts. Even with headache, I ignored it and told to myself that that pain was a reflection of my past, of what I had created for myself in the past and, on that day, I was in perfect health. The longer I stopped having thoughts about migraine, the more its synapses weakened. The more thoughts about perfect health, the more synapses appeared and the already existing ones strengthened. You need to do this: take the focus off the disease and put it in perfect health. Although it is difficult and sometimes discouraging, the effort is worth it because the prize is incomparable - PERFECT HEALTH! Below are some illustrative pictures of what was happening in my brain. Inclusion and exclusion.

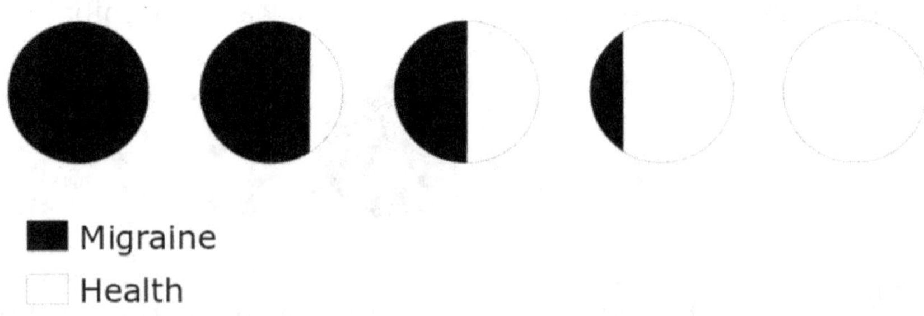

There were days I went through constant struggle against the 'status quo', my sickness self; but there were easier days, and over time, the easier days were getting more and more plentiful. My health was getting better. Not only that, the truth is that this change is so profound that it affects your whole life. You become the master of your brain and your whole life gets, with each passing day, better, happier, fuller. You learn that you are not your thoughts. You are not your feelings. You command them, you decide what to feel and what to think. The more you train, the easier it gets to achieve the results.

That's how I created a new standard of perfect health, replacing the old pattern of disease. As I said so many times before: if I could, you can too!

I will give another example in which I applied this method of inclusion/exclusion in my life, in a totally spontaneous, perhaps inspired way.

One of the migraine treatments I tried made me go into depression with anxiety and company crises. By the time I went into depression, I still did not have all the knowledge I have today, but what I had was enough to heal me. After a few months of depression, I started to do certain activities regardless of whether I wanted to do them or not. What I thought was my responsibility to do, I did. Even though I felt dead inside and totally hopeless. I started doing everything automatically and my instinct guided me to healing. I pushed all that lack of hope, sadness, defeatism, discouragement, weariness, etc., to a place far inside my mind and I locked everything there. It was as if I had made a deal with everything, with God and the universe: "okay, you're there, it sucks to live. I would probably have given up living if I did not have a young son, but... I have to keep living, so you'll stay there, in your place, and I'll pretend you do not exist." That done, I started to do things mechanically, without thinking about that all, lurking, threatening to throw myself down the drain. I felt all that, but I did not think about it. I decided not to have any internal dialogues about depression, injustice, or the famous "Why me?". I simply blocked that subject in my life and began to "live" regardless of that.

That's how I healed myself: I refrained from thinking about depression. I began to do everything that I have to do, with determination. I repeated incessantly to myself "I am very happy, I am very happy, I am very happy...". I said it day and night, I gave no room for other thoughts. Strenuous? Yes, for sure! But...!!! The alternative was worse. To feel constantly exhausted was even a blessing in view of that. I'll tell you something, I did not even notice the process, but one day, "all that" was gone.

I do not know exactly how long it took me to fully heal from depression. The improvement was gradual, but it did happen and there was a feeling in me that it was fast, maybe because I never believed I would or because I did not even know what I was doing. I just knew that I could not continue the way I was.

If you suffer from depression, decide now that you want to be happy and not, "I do not want to have depression anymore." Remember, "WE LIVE IN A UNIVERSE OF INCLUSION" and "YOU ARE NOT YOUR FEELINGS".

It's your choice. I healed myself! No medicine, and if I could, you can too. Feed the synapses of joy, love, and pleasure for life. Live one day at a time. Do not think about yesterday, or tomorrow. One step at a time. Do not think, "I do not believe I'm very happy and if I keep repeating this, it will not change my sad reality, it's stupid." That's where you go wrong, all your beliefs were created like this, with repetition. Remember:

"Your strongest beliefs had once been quiet thoughts."

When disbelief comes, think to yourself, "It is better to try to win than to grumble over a previous defeat". That is what I did and I do. It's my motto. It is always better to walk than to stand still. It's always best to try!

LIVING IN THE MATRIX

"ALL THINGS ARE SUBJECT TO INTERPRETATION.
WHATEVER INTERPRETATION PREVAILS IN A CERTAIN MOMENT,
IT IS A FUNCTION OF POWER AND NOT OF TRUTH."

FRIEDRICH NIETZSCHE

I think the best way to start this topic is by quoting the Allegory of the Cave by Plato.

"Imagine an underground cave where, from infancy, generation after generation, human beings are imprisoned. Their legs and necks are so fastened that they are forced to remain always in the same place and to look only forward, unable to turn their heads back and forth. The entrance to the cave allows some outside light to penetrate it, so that in the semi-darkness one can see what is happening inside.

The light comes from an immense fire that is outside the cave at the top of a hill. Between it and the prisoners - abroad, - there is an ascending path along which a wall was erected, as if it were the frontier part of a puppet stage. Along this wall, men carry statues of all kinds, with figures of human beings, animals, among other things.

Because of the light and the position occupied by it, the prisoners see on the wall at the bottom of the cave the shadows of the transported figurines, but without being able to see the statues themselves, or the men who carry them.

As they have never seen anything else, the prisoners think that the shadows seen are the things themselves. That is, they cannot know that they are shadows, nor can they know they are images, nor that there are other real human beings outside the cave. They also cannot know that they see because there is a light on the outside and they imagine that all possible luminosity is that which reigns in the cave.

What would happen if someone released the prisoners? What would a freed prisoner do? In the first place, he would look at the whole cave, see the other human beings, the wall, the statues, and the fire. Although pained by the years of immobility, he would begin to walk, going to the entrance of the cave and faced with the ascending path.

At first, he would be completely blind, because the fire was indeed the light of the sun, and he would be entirely blinded by it. Then, getting used to the light, he would see the men carrying the statues, and going on the way, he would see his own things, discovering that all his life he had seen is nothing but the shadow of images and that he is now contemplating his own reality.

Freed and knowledgeable of the world, the prisoner would return to the cave, be bewildered by the darkness, tell others what he saw and try to free them. But would the other prisoners believe it? Wouldn't they mock him?..."

The questions generated by this story are many, but the important thing here is to understand that most people live like these prisoners of Plato's story, trapped by the common sense of reality. The world out there is showing (it's actually screaming!) that all that reality "is not quite like that". There is more, much more than what we understand as reality. We are in the age of awakening. We are discovering the Matrix!

Learn and incorporate this: reality is not something that exists, it is something that you create!

"Our memories are not like fiction. They are fiction."

Jonah Lehrer

Do you think that Lehrer's quote is nonsense? It is not. If you take a memory of yourself and start counting it by modifying it, if you count it often, it will reach a point where you will not distinguish the original memory, you will believe what you are saying.

Not only that, think with me: the world already was flat, the Earth already was square, the sun has already revolved around the Earth. When men began to navigate the oceans, they were afraid of plummeting on the horizon. And the misperceptions of the human being do not stop there, they are innumerable.

Each of us experiences the world in a unique way. My green is not the same as yours. Our subconscious gives meaning to the events and stimuli we encounter by associating them with memories, beliefs, habits we create, and dictates how we relate to ourselves, others, and the world. This entire set of guidelines is formed over the years, especially up to the age of six, and is shaped by our family, religion, school, culture and past experiences. This targeting that the subconscious does is not even perceived by consciousness - you. You believe that whoever is in control of the decisions you make in your life is you. But it is not.

A vast amount of research has been conducted over the years about the subconscious mind. It was discovered that our brains begin to prepare for action a little more than a third of a second before we consciously decide to act. In other words, even when we "think" - we are aware - it is our subconscious mind that is actually making decisions for us.

Studies show as well that 95-99% of all our decisions, actions, emotions and behaviors come from the programming existing in our unconscious mind. This fact leaves us with only 1-5% of conscious decisions during the day, which by adding two plus two makes us realize that our subconscious mind is extremely more powerful than our conscious mind.

Do not despair though, it does not leave you with your hands and feet bound, at the mercy of this immense and unknown monster called the unconscious mind that guides your life. In fact, from the moment you become aware of this fact, this balance begins to change.

Remember that in one of the chapters above I told you that you should see yourself as three different parts? And that you should nominate these parts and deal with them in a specific way to each one? Do you see why? Your unconscious is Jack, the CEO of your body and your behavior. It manages your body because you are never there. You let him loose to do what he wants based on what he knows. But from the moment you start to pay attention to your body company, to appear every day and to determine your destiny, everything begins to change because, although Jack is much more inside everything that happens there than you, everything is yours, and, in the end, that's what matters. You are the boss.

Jack, your unconscious, is nothing but a supercomputer loaded with a database of programmed behaviors. Like any computer, you can reprogram it, install new software.

That makes you think, it raises a question; if what is out there is unique and only an interpretation of reality that my brain fabricate, can I induce my brain to see what I wish existed? Yes, you can. Using various lines of thought you come to that same conclusion. Let's talk about some.

LINE OF THOUGHT 1
IMAGINATION AND REALITY THE SAME THING

"IMAGINATION IS MORE IMPORTANT THAN KNOWLEDGE. FOR KNOWLEDGE IS LIMITED, WHEREAS IMAGINATION EMBRACES THE ENTIRE WORLD, STIMULATING PROGRESS, GIVING BIRTH TO EVOLUTION."

ALBERT EINSTEIN

Think about your dreams. How many times did you wake up shivering or crying, or feeling completely bad about something you dreamed about? It was just a dream, but for your brain it was real and all related chemicals, hormones, were released in your bloodstream and you feel every situation as if they were real.

Now, think about fears, even better, think about phobias. Did you get it? The reaction that someone has when dealing with any phobia is way stronger than the real threat.

Let's go a little further. Scientists have found that if you connect a person's brain to computers and scanners and are asked to look at certain objects, some areas of the brain will be activated. The cool thing about this research is what came after. Scientists then asked people to close their eyes and imagine the same object, and the same areas of the brain were activated, as if they were seeing the objects themselves. Is that not fantastic?!

And the researches do not stop there:

Students performed an experiment in which one group of individuals were asked to play piano, while another group were asked to imagine playing a piano. The reaction of the brain among those who only imagined was the same observed in those who in reality played the instrument.

A study done at the University of Ohio shows that being quiet while thinking about exercise can make us stronger. Brian Clark and his colleagues recruited 29 volunteers and wrapped their wrists with plaster for a whole month. For 11 minutes a day, 5 days a week, half the volunteers sat completely still and concentrated all their mental effort on pretending to flex their muscles. When the plasters were removed, the volunteers who did mental exercises had wrist muscles twice as strong as those who had not done anything.

What does this mean in practical terms? Chemicals reactions occur in your body independent of being based on what is called reality or not. How to use this knowledge? Pretend you have/is all you want to have or be. Behave yourself, dress and speak as the person you would like to be. If you want to become more confident, steady your chest, straighten your posture and walk as if the world were yours, the famous superhero attitude! If you want to lose weight, instead of looking in the mirror always and seeing what you do not like, create your imaginary mirror in your head, seeing yourself as you would like to be. Take a portrait of you and paste it into the body you would like to have and always keep it in sight. Re-create and pretend. It will become reality.

LINE OF THOUGHT 2
EVERYTHING IS ENERGY

"THE ATOMS OR ELEMENTARY PARTICLES
THEMSELVES ARE NOT REAL; THEY FORM A WORLD OF POTENTIALITIES OR
POSSIBILITIES RATHER THAN ONE OF THINGS OR FACTS."

WERNER HEISENBERG

Let's think in quantum terms...

Quantum physics says that as you delve deeper into the operation of the atoms, you realize that there is nothing there – just waves of energy. An atom is literally an invisible force field, a kind of miniature tornado, which emits waves of energy.

These waves of energy can be measured and their effects seen, but they are not a material reality. They have no substance because they are energy.

In the last century Einstein already spoke about this, with his formula $E=mc^2$. In practical terms what this formula brings us is that matter is nothing more than condensed energy and vice versa. Matter and energy are the different faces of the same coin. With this, you begin to see that you really know nothing of the world you live in, that what is called reality is something much more complex and ephemeral than you might imagine. You also realize the world of possibilities that it brings to you.

Have you seen any video explaining the double-slit experience? You must see. This video below is very explanatory and easy to understand:

https://www.youtube.com/watch?v=btImof4nyzo

In the basic version of this double-slit experiment, single particles, such as photons, pass one at a time through a screen containing two slits. If one of the paths is monitored, a photon apparently passes through a slit or another, and no interference will be seen. On the other hand, if neither is monitored, a photon will appear through both slits simultaneously before interfering with itself, acting like a wave.

Anyway, what is important to us is what conclusion the researchers came up with in this experiment. This experiment showed that what we call "matter", like electrons, somehow combines particle and wave characteristics. When the experiment happens without an observer, or without something to measure, the electrons behave as waves and interfere with each other, and when there is an observer, the behavior of the electrons is totally different, they behave like particles, producing two marks on the wall.

In practical terms the double-slit experience shows us that we live in a field of potentialities determined by ourselves, not in a static, predetermined world. The implications of this discovery are incredible and immeasurable, for the only possible conclusion that the researchers have reached is that all reality is a matter of how we perceive and measure it. This measurement is what ultimately composes reality and not the opposite. This shakes the foundations of an objective reality and places us not as spectators, but as a fundamental creator of reality.

If everything is energy and I can, through my attention, modify the world around me, what can I do in practical terms? Everything! You just need to train. Over time you're getting good at manipulating everything around you.

LINE OF THOUGHT 3

"AS A MAN THINKETH, SO HE IS."

PROVERBS 23: 7

In religious terms? Jesus was a great propagator of the concept of potentialities field. It's there in the Bible for anyone who wants to read.

"SO I SAY TO YOU: ASK AND IT WILL BE GIVEN TO YOU; SEEK AND YOU WILL FIND; KNOCK AND THE DOOR WILL BE OPENED TO YOU. FOR EVERYONE WHO ASKS RECEIVES; THE ONE WHO SEEKS FINDS; AND TO THE ONE WHO KNOCKS, THE DOOR WILL BE OPENED."
LUKE 11: 9,10

"IF YOU BELIEVE, YOU WILL RECEIVE WHATEVER YOU ASK FOR IN PRAYER."
MATTHEW 21:22

"BECAUSE YOU HAVE SO LITTLE FAITH. TRULY I TELL YOU, IF YOU HAVE FAITH AS SMALL AS A MUSTARD SEED, YOU CAN SAY TO THIS MOUNTAIN, 'MOVE FROM HERE TO THERE,' AND IT WILL MOVE. NOTHING WILL BE IMPOSSIBLE FOR YOU."
MATTHEW 17:20

"JUST THEN A WOMAN WHO HAD BEEN SUBJECT TO BLEEDING FOR TWELVE YEARS CAME UP BEHIND HIM AND TOUCHED THE EDGE OF HIS CLOAK. SHE SAID TO HERSELF, "IF I ONLY TOUCH HIS CLOAK, I WILL BE HEALED." JESUS TURNED AND SAW HER. "TAKE HEART, DAUGHTER," HE SAID, "YOUR FAITH HAS HEALED YOU." AND THE WOMAN WAS HEALED AT THAT MOMENT."
MATTHEW 9: 21-22

"WHEN HE HAD GONE INDOORS, THE BLIND MEN CAME TO HIM, AND HE ASKED THEM, "DO YOU BELIEVE THAT I AM ABLE TO DO THIS?"
"YES, LORD," THEY REPLIED.
THEN HE TOUCHED THEIR EYES AND SAID, "ACCORDING TO YOUR FAITH LET IT BE DONE TO YOU." AND THEIR SIGHT WAS RESTORED..."
MATTHEW 9:28-30

"TRULY I TELL YOU, IF ANYONE SAYS TO THIS MOUNTAIN, 'GO, THROW YOURSELF INTO THE SEA,' AND DOES NOT DOUBT IN THEIR HEART BUT BELIEVES THAT WHAT THEY SAY WILL HAPPEN, IT WILL BE DONE FOR THEM. THEREFORE, I TELL YOU, WHATEVER YOU ASK FOR IN PRAYER, BELIEVE THAT YOU HAVE RECEIVED IT, AND IT WILL BE YOURS..."
MARK 11:23-24

"THAT DAY WHEN EVENING CAME, HE SAID TO HIS DISCIPLES, "LET US GO OVER TO THE OTHER SIDE." LEAVING THE CROWD BEHIND, THEY TOOK HIM ALONG, JUST AS HE WAS, IN THE BOAT. THERE WERE ALSO OTHER BOATS WITH HIM. A FURIOUS SQUALL CAME UP, AND THE WAVES BROKE OVER THE BOAT, SO THAT IT WAS NEARLY SWAMPED. JESUS WAS IN THE STERN, SLEEPING ON A CUSHION. THE DISCIPLES WOKE HIM AND SAID TO HIM, "TEACHER, DON'T YOU CARE IF WE DROWN?" HE GOT UP, REBUKED THE WIND AND SAID TO THE WAVES, "QUIET! BE STILL!" THEN THE WIND DIED DOWN AND IT WAS COMPLETELY CALM. HE SAID TO HIS DISCIPLES, "WHY ARE YOU SO AFRAID? DO YOU STILL HAVE NO FAITH?"
MARK 4:35

Whoever has actually read the Bible knows that Jesus always teaches us that we live in a world of possibilities, teaches us that whatever we want, if we have faith, we will receive. He multiplied food, made the blind see, made the paralyzed walk again, resurrected people, turned water into wine and the only thing he asked of the men is that they had faith in their hearts.

Block 3

"Knowing others is intelligence; knowing yourself is true wisdom. Mastering others is strength; mastering yourself is true power."

Lao Tzu

Techniques and Natural Alternatives

There are several techniques that can help you in difficult times and others which you should incorporate into your routine, and do not use the 'bullshit' (sorry the expression) of the "timeless". Time is made, time is prioritized. There is no lack of time. There is only your inability to deal with it. What you should do is learn how to manage your time, there are a lot of books on the subject. But even then, you still must decide what is important to you, what you should to incorporate in your routine to achieve your goals. A tip that I use is doing every day what I want to introduce/keep in my daily activities, even just a little. If you are committed to doing every day, you cut off excuses like: I'll do it tomorrow/Monday/next week. Did you get it?

Let's take an example - meditation. Meditation is that kind of activity you should keep doing every day, so... I do it every day (not tomorrow, even on weekends!) even when the time runs out, I sit or lay and meditate for 5 minutes at least. Everyone has 5 minutes. It's just a matter of decision. Decide, I'll do and I'll do every day.

Here are some natural alternatives and techniques I recommend:

- Meditation;

- EFT;

- Past-Life Therapy;

- Bowling Ball Syndrome;

- Isochronic and binaural sounds;

-   Use a bracelet with magnetic therapy;

-   Sunlight exposure;

-   Read;

-   Have contact with nature;

-   Practice exercises;

-   Reiki;

-   Flowers Therapy like Bach, California, Bush and Minas.

All these techniques and natural alternatives are worth trying in pursuit of perfect health. Some will work for you and some will not. Below I comment on some.

MEDITATION

The first technique I recommend is to meditate and this is one that you should incorporate into your routine.

Let's start talking about meditation, first of all you should demystify and stop labeling it. I have already realized that most people have the tendency to mystify or demean the practice of meditation by putting it in the exoteric zone. Overcome this, meditating is super easy and the benefits of meditation has already been proven by science through studies using MRI and CAT scan so that even the incredibly skeptics cannot question it efficacy.

Some of the things that science has proven: meditation causes physical changes in the brain, it increases the activity of the anterior cingulate cortex (area attached to attention and concentration), the prefrontal cortex (connected to motor coordination), and the hippocampus, increasing the volume of the gray matter. It also acts on the amygdala, which regulates emotions and, when triggered, accelerates the functioning of the hypothalamus, related to the sensation of relaxation. Meditation upturn your whole brain.

Several studies have shown that the practice of meditation helps to reduce depression, targeting this problem in its most common triggers such as stress, anxiety and fears. If you think that depression has increased among the world population over the last few years and becoming more and more a major health issue, meditating can be an easy and effective way of prevention and cure.

According to Dr. John W. Denninger, director of research at the Benson-Henry Institute for Mind Body Medicine at Harvard-affiliated Massachusetts General Hospital: "Meditation trains the brain to achieve sustained focus, and to return to that focus when negative thinking, emotions, and physical sensations intrude -which happens a lot when you feel stressed and anxious".

I will list some of the many benefits that this practice brings, in simpler terms:

- Reduction of stress;

- Improvement of the cardiovascular system;

- Improvement in sleep quality;

- Improvement of depression and anxiety;

- Relief of pain and decreased frequency of migraines;

- Enhanced immune system;

- Improved concentration;

- Reverses aging.

Above all, meditation improves well-being. Want something better than feeling at peace, feeling good about yourself, focused? That's the best meditation can bring, in my opinion.

As for how to meditate, easy topic, choose the method you prefer, because another thing that science has proven is that all forms of meditation provoke similar results. Before exposing some methods, I want to tell you some simple and uncomplicated guidelines that I have learned throughout my more than 20 years of meditation. You can meditate in any way, lying down, sitting, reclining, it does not matter, in any position you will feel the benefits of meditation. What matters is that you quiet your mind, diminish the eternal buzz that most people carry inside their heads, "Did I leave the fire on?, Did I turn on the car alarm?, Will this shirt be adequate?, I cannot remember the name of this song." and so on. Can you imagine how exhausting it must be for your brain?! Having to command the whole body machine - breathe in, breathe out, beat, contract, strange particle coming in, warm up, shiver - and besides, you are there, with that endless twist rolling on your head? No wonder most people today are stressed out. But it is possible to cease those buzzings - which are just automatic responses that you have become accustomed to have - through meditation.

That is precisely the focus of meditation, to diminish the thoughts that keep you from living life fully. Most of the time, these thoughts are useless and repetitive, reaffirming our beliefs and paradigms, bringing underlying feelings that make us anxious, frustrated, afraid. This heap of thought makes us lose the focus of the present moment. Which is why we often eat without tasting our food, or we look at a person without really seeing them.

In short, to meditate is nothing but to distance yourself from this mental cacophony, giving room for your higher mind to breathe. Observe the murmur, but do not partake in it, and as you do it, it will diminish, and keep diminishing. You begin to see things more clearly, have your attention more focused on what you are doing rather than divided between what you do and the unceasing nonsense speech in your mind.

"My meditation is simple.

It does not require any complex practice.

It's simple. Sing. dance.

Sitting silently."

Osho

Another thing, do not be fooled by the flourishing that some people tend to do when it comes to meditation. Meditation is simple and easy, and any time is better than none, as I always say. Start with 5 minutes a day, do not commit too much, commit to doing 5 minutes every day and if it happens to be able to do more, great, even better. When you want to acquire a new habit, the best way is with goals that you are sure you will be able to fulfill, this avoids frustration and the sense of failure, the sense of I cannot. A habit is formed by constancy and repetition. Also, do not tell yourself: "meditation is not for me, I cannot stop thinking". In the beginning no one can really silent his mind. It is the training that gives you this ability and, to get good at anything... the only way is training.

So, choose the method that makes you more comfortable and go for it. Here are some:

- **Mindfulness**: This method is the most talked at the moment. It is nothing else than simply focusing on the present moment, observing what is happening to you, in your reality, seeing your thoughts, emotions, but without judging them, without making emotional evaluations or reacting automatically.

Put yourself in a comfortable position and begin by paying attention to your breathing, feeling the air coming in, expanding your abdomen, then exhaling. Let your mind go away from the outside world, ceasing to hear external noises. Feel the peace invading your body and your mind. If your thoughts persist to appear, do not fight against them, do not focus on them, move away.

- **Visualization**: In visualization the intention is to use only one sense, the vision, which is usually the strongest sense of most people, causing everything else to dissipate and blur. Choose an image that brings you well-being; a child running on a sunny green field, the sea, a field of flowers, it does not matter, as long as it inspires good feelings. Focus your gaze on this image as you breathe in and breathe out deeply. You can also imagine yourself sitting at the bottom of a pool, paying attention to the balls of air that flow out from your nose toward the surface. You can focus on anything, even a hole in the wall, the goal is to decrease your conscious activity. If your view blurs, no problem, focus again on what you've chosen as your view object.

- **Thematic meditation**: Focus on a high feeling like love, peace, faith, compassion, happiness, there are many to choose. Choose what inspires you the most and think about it. Repeat for yourself the word and let the images related to the subject you choose come up in your mind. It's not something like by thinking about love and remembering the person who betrayed you, whom you cannot trust anymore, etc. You will think about love from a high perspective, above human meanness.

Sometimes, when time is short, or simply because I want to rescue that sense of well-being that meditation brings, I sit or lie, depending on where I am, and I watch the sky, the clouds passing through, forget all the rest and let all that blue come into me. The blue sky always brings a sense of peace, at least to me. Or I watch a big tree, a pretty lawn. This is meditating too!

You can also do a guided meditation if you prefer. There are many of them, with several different approaches. Find what works for you, and as I've said countless times, do not overcharge yourself, just persist.

Past Life Therapy

"There are things known and there are things unknown, and in between are the doors of perception."

Aldous Huxley

Regression to past lives is still a very controversial subject, and I will not get into that discussion, it's not worth it. From a very young age I learned to stop asking myself, "is this real or not?". My philosophy has always been: does it work? If so, the rest is just story. I do not care what the various religions say about it, or the doctors, or the charlatans. I do not care if it's in my head or if it's a real memory. The only thing that matters to me is if it works, if it brings results. And I advise all people to have the same policy on various subjects related to the human mind. As Shakespeare said, "There are more things in heaven and earth. Than are dreamt of in your philosophy." So, never limit your reality by the borders of contemporary human knowledge.

Past life regression did not help me in curing chronic pain, but I think it worthwhile to expose this technique because it helped me in numerous other problems, among them, in curing asthma, another chronic illness. I was born with asthma, and when I remember that, I always think, "My poor parents, having a child with a chronic illness that has no cure (it does not have a traditional cure, I mean) must have been an emotionally terrible thing to live with". But getting back to the subject, healing myself from asthma was almost an accident. Before I explain how this happened I'll tell you when I first met the past-life therapy.

I've always been a voracious reader, the kind who reads almost everything. Even my life story has contributed to this habit, sick child, frequently in bed with parents that enjoy reading?! Although my body was often stuck, my mind could travel wherever the book took me.

My first contact with the subject "regression" was through the books of Lobsang Rampa, which did not encourage the practice at all. It was only later, when "Many Lives, Many Masters" (Brian Weiss) fell into my hands that I began to practice it. This book marked me deeply, opened up a huge range of possibilities for me, and in addition, I loved the non-religious approach on the subject. After that, I read two others by the same author, Only love is real and Through Time into Healing, which taught me how to regress. I thought back then that I could solve any problem in my life by regressing. It's not entirely so, there are problems that simply do not originate from a past life, so, of course, you cannot solve them using regression.

For a long time, I was always regressing and I had two regressions which, in my opinion, were the reason I got cured of asthma. In one of them I was a boy who was caught stealing in the Alexandria market and was trapped in a cell below ground level. In this cell there was only a crack on the top to get air. The memory was very bad. I think, since I was very young, having been trapped in a place that looked like a hole in the ground was very traumatic. I was suffocating inside. In the other memory I died from drowning in the sea. After these two regressions I never had any asthma attack. Does it look like a miracle? Yes, it does, but it happened to me. As I said above, I did not care if it was a memory of past lives or something of my mind, I got cured of a disease that had been suffering since I was born. That's what matters and will always matter - results.

It may be that your healing is also in this practice or it may not be, what matters is that if there is a chance for healing, it is worth trying.

A curiosity that happened to me related to past lives that, although not related to the subject of this book, I find interesting to tell is one that occurred the first time I went to France. From the first night I slept there, I began to have a dream so vivid and so intense that I got out of bed desperate, most of the time screaming, trying to leave the place where I was, as if I still in my dream, until my husband got me back to reality, which every time took a while. It was always the same nightmare. I was underground in a subway station and the walls were falling on top of me and I became desperate because nobody knew I was there. I knew in my dream that the second great war was happening. The strange thing is that I never had that kind of nightmare, as soon as I arrived in England the nightmare stopped, and when I returned to Paris to leave for Brazil, they returned. On another occasion I went to Europe, I traveled from Italy to Switzerland through the Alps, passing through France and entering Switzerland through Geneva, on the nights I spent in French territory I experienced the same nightmares I had the first time I went there. Super strange, isn't it? And totally without explanation. But you cannot say it's a coincidence, right? I think this experience I went through is one of those things that proves that there is so much more than we can fully understand.

To help start the practice or understand more, I recommend Brian Weiss's books. He has a book with a guided regression audio, Mirrors of time. There is also a guided meditation that I have already practiced a lot too. I think it's a good start, and once the technique is mastered, they are no longer needed. But the internet is a very large field of resources, it is up to each one to seek out the most appropriate form for themselves.

EMOTIONAL FREEDOM TECHNIQUES

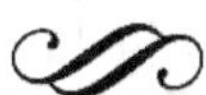

In the short time since Emotional Freedom Techniques (EFT) inception, in 90`s, it has provided thousands of people relief for a variety of problems and conditions, often in a surprisingly fast time and after long and painful periods of seeking a cure. The diversity of successful treatments ranges from trauma and phobias to behavioral patterns of self-sabotage, anxiety, depression, addictions, physical illnesses, chronic pain, to name a few. It's worth a try, I recommend it.

It uses the same principles of acupuncture to break energetic blockages in the body, considered the origin of the most diverse problems, either physical or emotional. That is a simplistic description, but it is not my intention in this book to make anyone an EFT expert, but rather to present the tools I used in my healing and personal development process. A lot of researches have been done and others are underway regarding the effectiveness of this technique. There is plenty of material available on the internet for those who wish to delve into the subject.

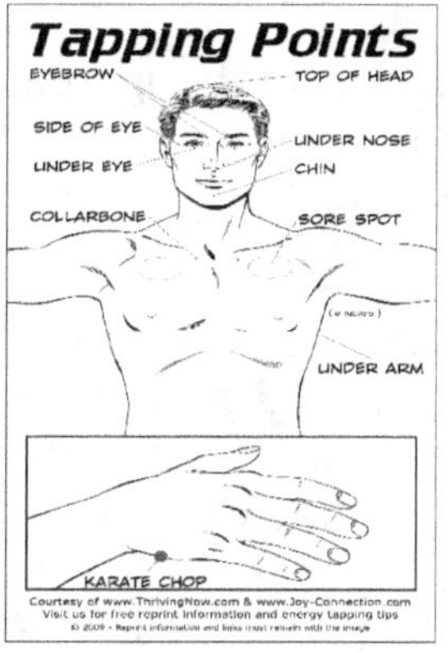

How EFT works? There is a sequence of points on the body

where you must tap lightly a couple of times while talking about the problem you want to solve. The picture above shows the EFT points.

You will start with the Karate chop and the most common sequence after is eyebrow, side of eye, under eye, under nose, chin, collarbone, under arm, top of head and go on again and again.

I will try to describe how it is done, but it is much easier to watch a video. You identify the problem you want to solve. It can be anxiety, pain, a guilt that you carry with you that makes you feel bad. You think about the problem, even if it brings you discomfort. In fact, the ideal is that you feel the discomfort because the more intensely you feel your problem, the more EFT will produce result. Take a sheet of paper and write short sentences that summarize your problem for you to use during EFT.

On a scale of 0 to 10, decide the intensity that this problem affects you and write it down, along with the sentences. Do not waste much time on it, it's just a measurement, something to compare before and after.

Usually you start knocking on the karate point with a phrase that says that even if you have this problem, you love and accept yourself. You hit the karate spot while repeating the phrase three times.

To pain: "Even if I feel this pain ... (in the head, in the back, in the legs, etc.), I love and accept myself deeply and completely."

To fears: "Even though I feel all this fear, panic of ... (flying, heights, spider, etc.), I love and accept myself just the way I am and I choose to accept these feelings and set myself free"

To forgive yourself: "Even though part of me feels that I deserve this shame and it is necessary to prevent me from making such mistakes in the future, I'm ready to let go of this feeling, and set myself free."

Phrases can be written in many ways, you just need to speak your problem and make an affirmation of acceptance. Then you keep tapping the EFT points, speaking the phrases you noted in the preparation or just repeating the problem, if you want to be very direct. I often did EFT just repeating the phrase "this headache, this headache". Which is very specific and localized, helping to relieve the pain.

Important: It is essential that the phrases are negative or make you feel the problem because the goal is to feel the negative energy related to the problem so EFT can clear that energy from your body.

The easiest way to learn EFT is by doing it. Go to YouTube, watch some videos about the technique and quickly you can master the technique, which is very simple. Like meditation, there is no difficulty in doing EFT, I have always done it on my own and I have had excellent results.

Bowling Ball Syndrome

This syndrome occurs when the sphenoid bone (the keystone of your cranium) is not in its appropriate place. When the sphenoid bone is moved, the other bones will follow it to compensate the body balance, and by doing this it will generate a constant tension throughout the body. This permanent tension can cause innumerous problems such as migraine, back pain, allergies, temporomandibular joint (TMJ) syndrome, etc.

This misalignment can be caused by injuries in the skull or neck – generally occurred during childhood.

Just to clarify, the name of this syndrome is based on the fact that the head weighs approximately as much as a bowling ball.

In your book "Healing is voltage" (you should read), Dr. Tennant says –"Almost everyone suffering from chronic illness has the bowling ball syndrome. One of the amazing things that happens when you correct it is that it balances the sympathetic and parasympathetic system. ...This allows you to enter 'parasympathetic-on' with the ability to have normal digestion, sleep better and heal."

There are several manual ways to solve this problem, but Dr. Tennant has created an instrument called biomodulator that by applying electrical stimulation in determined points of the neck, it can correct the abnormal position of the skull and cervical vertebrae. In just a few minutes.

BRAINWAVES

"IF YOU ARE DEPRESSED, YOU ARE LIVING IN THE PAST.
IF YOU ARE ANXIOUS, YOU ARE LIVING IN THE FUTURE.
IF YOU ARE AT PEACE, YOU ARE LIVING IN THE PRESENT."

LAO TZU

I'll summarize what brainwaves are before I explain how to use them. As you must know, the brain is an electrochemical organ, which means that if you connect enough wires to your scalp, you can even turn on a light bulb. The electrical communication happens through neurons, which are specialized brain cells responsible for transmitting information through the body and they do it chemically and electrically. The electrical activity emanating from these communications between neurons is measured in the form of brain waves. Until now, five brain waves have been measured: Gamma, Beta, Alpha, Theta and Delta. And each of them is associated with a specific type of task and mental state.

Delta: In general, Delta waves are generated when the person is in a deep sleep but not dreaming or in a very deep meditative state.

Theta: Theta waves are related to vivid dreams, intuition and creativity. They also appear when the person is in deep meditation.

Alpha: Alpha waves support general mental coordination, calmness, attention, mind/body integration and learning.

Beta: Beta waves dominate our normal state of consciousness. We're in beta most of the time when we're awake. It is present when we are attentive, involved in solving problems.

Gamma: Gamma waves are the least known. They are difficult to measure by instruments normally used for this purpose. Gamma waves are related to elevated mental states of great joy, universal love and spiritual connection.

You must be wondering, "What's all this got to do with this book, with me?" I'll explain. Just as your mental state produces certain brain waves, you can too do the reverse, use sounds to produce a particular brain wave, and thus change the state in which you are. I'll explain better. You are restless, nervous, do not know how to solve a problem, etc. Rather than stress yourself over the subject you can quietly sit down somewhere, plug in your headphones and hear binaural beats and isochronic sounds to induce the production of alpha waves that, as you read above, is the wave of tranquility. Can you do that? Yes. There is a lot of material on the internet, just search on YouTube; including some sounds directly focused on pain relief.

I use daily binaural and isochronic sounds with subliminal messages to modify or emphasize a specific thought pattern. I think it's fantastic how it really works. As you know, most of your habits were created in the first seven years of your life and in these early years your mind function in theta waves, which are the subconscious mind change waves. To change a habit, you have two ways: repeat, repeat and repeat or download a new program through binaural and isochronic sounds with subliminal messages.

I highly recommend listening to it.

What I Did At The Beginning!

As I said in the beginning of this book, the first thing I did was take a decision. I decided! Without a "but" after. I decided that no matter how bad /hard/discouraging it was, I would persevere. I had a goal – perfect health – and I was going to reach it. I took that real leap of faith, even though I did not completely believe it. I decided that my beliefs had nothing to do with reaching my goal, they will not interfere anymore. My life was horrible, and with each passing year I was getting worse. I had to do something. Several books and videos I read said that my whole life was a product of what I thought and even if I could not understand or find my thoughts of having "headache", I decided that I would, EVEN WITHOUT BELIEVE, see if there was a sense in all this chat about the law of attraction. I cut the migraine/headache/illness issue out of my life. Of course, everything was a process. It was not magic. The change was gradual and sometimes, when the discouragement and pain came up, I thought I would never really have perfect health. But I got it. In those moments, I pushed all those "old" thoughts aside and did anything to distract myself such as watching tv series that I loved or read a good book. This is a tip: create your escapes, things you enjoy doing, books and funny movies, tv series, etc., so you will have something to put your mind out of difficulties.

After deciding, I cut out all the medicines I was taking. Concomitantly, I started taking omega 3, iodine, vitamin B2, vitamin B6, magnesium and turmeric. I drank ginger tea and mustard seed tea every day. Another mix I did when I felt pain was to add a shallow teaspoon of maca with a generous pinch of ginger powder in a glass of water and drink.

TEA RECIPE:

Ginger tea:

Cut ±5cm of ginger root and half large lemon in slices. Put everything in a cup, add ½ teaspoon of cinnamon. Pour boiling water and leave to brew for 10 minutes. Add honey and drink.

Note: This tea is amazing. When I started drinking it, I had a rhinitis bothering me for a while. After one month I realized that the rhinitis was gone. It never came back because I still drink the tea almost every day.

Mustard Seed Tea:

Mix 1 tablespoon of mustard seed and the same amount of fennel seed in a cup. Add boiling water and leave to infuse for 10 minutes. Then sprinkle some cinnamon and drink.

My natural alternatives to controlling or ending pain at that time were these teas. Sometimes taking a flat teaspoon of baking soda with water or citrus juice helped. When the pain started to bother me a lot, I took a super slow bath, being underwater decreased the pain. I took turmeric with magnesium. Another alternative is getting a thin cloth, putting two ice blocks in it and then tying it on the forehead (as a ninja) with the ice touching through the cloth on the region between the eyes. It works wonders when you are in pain. At first it hurts, but then it passes and it takes nausea away. Decreasing pain. Another natural alternative that I used to use was EFT.

I also imposed the rule of doing exercise every day, 20 minutes minimum, usually a stationary bicycle, because it is the kind of physical activity you can do no matter the weather. You can work out hard or light and moreover, if you are the type that needs an extra stimulus to do exercise, you can always tune in to your favorite program on the television or read an interesting book. 20 minutes will pass super-fast.

I studied and studied. Always. Books and videos appeared to me. Clearly, I was being guided to achieve what I desired, to have perfect health. What happened as a result was that the changes taking place in my paradigms affected my way of acting and my new way of acting reinforced my new thoughts and I began to have a better life in every aspect of it.

Nowadays, I continue with part of these supplements and added others. I try to follow the ketogenic diet, but I'm not that kind of paranoid, all-or-nothing type. If I want to eat something, I'll eat it. I do not deprive myself, I'm just selective. I try to eat organic foods whenever possible and it's extremely rare that I consume gluten or fried foods. Many people say that consuming organic food is impossible due to the exorbitant prices. I'll tell you what, you have no idea how much I spent on medicines every month. The choice is yours as well. Like everything else in life, it's a matter of priorities, and in my opinion, there's nothing more important than being healthy. Today, after all these changes I have incorporated, my health is excellent. I am super active and full of energy, and I am extremely grateful for everything I have achieved. When I look at myself and see who I am now, and who I was, it even looks like a miracle!

I continue studying, always seeking knowledge that makes me evolve in every way. With each passing day, it is easier for me to manipulate the field of potentialities. As a last advice, what I can tell you is that IT ONLY DEPENDS ON YOU!

JUST TO REMEMBER:

AT THE END OF THIS MOVIE WE DIE. SO LIVE, DANCE, SING, SHOUT, SMILE, SPREAD LOVE, BE FREE, ENJOY EVERY MOMENT OF YOUR LIFE!

UNKNOWN AUTHOR